SILVER SCARS

SILVER SCARS

SARAH KRIVOS

Copyright © 2026 by Sarah Krivos

All rights reserved. No part of this book may be reproduced in any manner whatsoever without written permission except in the case of brief quotations embodied in critical articles and reviews.

ISBN 979-8-9940889-0-6
Library of Congress Cataloging-in-Publication Data is available on request.

First Printing, 2026
Reveal Publishing
Waukesha, WI

linkedin.com/in/sarahkrivos

For all of you battling an invisible disease. **I see you.**

The world breaks everyone and afterward many are strong at the broken places.

Ernest Hemingway, *A Farewell to Arms*

CHAPTER 1

Champagne Supernova

SEPTEMBER 4, 2017

"I think I'm dying, and I don't know why." These are the words I utter out of desperation to my unsuspecting husband, Dan, the night before our eldest daughter, Everly, begins 4K.

A chilled bottle of Mumm Napa Brut Rosé is nestled in a silver ice bucket, beads of condensation slowly forming on the outside, two beautiful crystal champagne flutes sitting next to it on the bathtub ledge. The oversized ivory whirlpool tub is almost filled to the top. Steam rises as eucalyptus Epsom salts dissolve and mix with the lavender bubble bath to create a fragrant spa-like atmosphere. Scalding-hot water tenderly burns our toes and tinges our cheeks pink with warmth as we slowly sink and relax into the deep tub.

We adopted our signature champagne bath ritual early on in our relationship, and it has evolved into a safe space where we talk, reconnect with one another as partners instead of as parents, and remember why we chose each other to venture through this crazy life together. Friends and family have enviously and playfully mocked us for years about this guilty pleasure, but some of our best conversations have occurred during a champs bath.

This one feels different, though, a last hurrah and final goodbye to summer mixed with an undercurrent of something dark and shadowy I can't quite pinpoint but that weighs heavily on my entire being.

After drying off, I sit on the side of the tub, dressed in a large, flowing, powder-blue-and-white-striped sleep shirt, similar to the one that Mom used to wear before she got sick. I feel drunk and woozy. It doesn't make sense that I am so inebriated after only two glasses of champagne, but it certainly makes it easier to articulate myself to Dan without the usual constraints of soberness. Alcohol has slowly become a third party in our marriage this summer, and now it provides me with the courage to finally give voice to the desolation that has been growing inside of me for the past nine months. I watch as a traffic jam of filmy soap bubbles congregates around the drain, each bubble trying to be the first one to make its way out of the tub, like impatient children jostling each other to win the coveted first place in line.

"Well, maybe you should go see another doctor," Dan says in an exasperated voice as he slightly rolls his eyes in annoyance. "I don't understand why you've changed so much. You're a completely different person lately, and I don't even know who you are anymore. If you really feel that bad, then do something about it."

The underlying tension that has been simmering between us all year long is coming to a head. His tone is sharper than usual, abrupt, his customary patience worn thin from the recent months of my escalating fatigue, moodiness, and irritability. Our words are forced, robotic. Resentment and misunderstanding crackle between us like electric wires.

Wet, fat, salty droplets land on the blue stripe of my sleep shirt and turn it navy. I stare at the spot intently so I don't have to look him directly in the eyes.

"I don't know what's going on. I feel terrible all day, every day, from the moment I open my eyes to the time I lie down in bed. I am so exhausted, but I haven't been able to sleep in months. Something is wrong with me. I'm scared. I don't know where to turn for help, and I'm terrified our kids are going to be motherless soon."

I cannot understand his obliviousness to the pain and torture I have been enduring. Then again, how could anyone possibly understand the depths of hell I have descended into when I still look so normal, so like me on the outside? I have become a master of forgery, perfecting the sleight-of-hand magic trick that hides the counterfeit life I am truly living. I play the part of doting stay-at-home, work-from-home housewife and mother so well that even I start believing my own bullshit façade and convince myself that I am not sick. The pictures I post on my Facebook page are the diametrical opposite of what is occurring inside of me. "Oh, look at this beautiful snapshot of my family smiling nonchalantly, looking at the camera but not posing. We are all happy and healthy, covered in glitter and unicorn fairy dust." And then five seconds later I'm snapping at Dan or the kids because they glance at me the wrong way.

I break down, sobbing, devastated that I must acknowledge the seriousness that something is undeniably wrong with me. Dan stalks out of the bathroom, slams the door harder than necessary, and stomps downstairs. An involuntary guttural sound emanates from the back of my throat. The brokenness inside is escaping, shattering me into something unrecognizable. I am terrified. Little do I know this is only the beginning.

CHAPTER 2

Thanks for the Memories

1985

My brothers and I throw open the back door of our family's rambling one-story ranch home and run with reckless abandon, scampering across our sprawling Wisconsin backyard to the dilapidated swing set bordering the rest of our heavily wooded property. The hard plastic seat of the red swing has faded to a light pink, and the cheap rubber tubes covering the links of the metal handles dried out years ago, disintegrating completely and turning to dust, leaving our small hands burgundy and covered in rust.

We pump our small legs as fast as possible and think that if we can only get the slightest bit higher, we will surely touch the sky and kiss the clouds. The silver steel slide absorbs the sun's heat on these long summer days, and it scorches our skin and burns our legs to a pink cotton-candy crisp. The rickety blue teeter-totter becomes a horse that my brothers try to throw me off of, landing as hard as they can on the ground while I'm up in the air on the other side. My shrill shrieks do little to deter their devious ways and only encourage their mischievous behavior.

The afternoon light fades quickly, and the amber glow filtering through the leaves of the forest suddenly turns foreboding. The branches of the trees that welcomed us with open arms just an hour ago now seem threatening, pointing at us critically with long, skinny, gnarled fingers, forcing us abruptly toward the safety and comfort of the house. We race each other back to the house, stampede through the living room, and skid to a halt on the yellowing linoleum floor of the kitchen where our mother hollers, "Go wash your hands!"

After rinsing our hands with a few droplets of water and even less soap, we scarf down our dinner of hot dogs and mac 'n' cheese, arguing over who won the race back to the house—none of us realizing that my petite five-year-old body just became the main entrée for a tiny bloodsucker.

The tick waited patiently on the green blade of overgrown grass for days, hunting, stalking, ready for its unsuspecting prey to recklessly wander past. Its eight legs were covered in short, spiny hairs that ended with tiny, curved claws. Between the two claws was a small, sticky pad to assist it in locating, grasping, and crawling onto its innocent host—me. Unnoticed, it stealthily made its way from my ankle to the top of my strawberry-blonde head, where it finally declared victory and burrowed into my scalp.

At school several days later, I sit on the story carpet and listen, mesmerized, to Mrs. Bernstein read *Corduroy* and pray that the teddy bear will find his missing button as well as a home. Reaching up to scratch my head, I feel a foreign object, as though the eraser from the top of a pencil has gotten mysteriously stuck there. I try pulling it, the way you pick at an annoying scab before it's ready to fall off, but it's firmly rooted in place. Shrugging nonchalantly and thinking nothing further of it, I put my hand back in my lap and smile happily when I hear that Corduroy has found his forever home with a loving little girl.

Bounding down the steps of the bright-yellow school bus that afternoon, I run into my mother's warm embrace and tell her all about the teddy bear with the missing button before casually mentioning the bump on my head. A highly respected radiologist, Mom has surely seen her fair share of grotesque and disturbing medical things, so I am rightfully scared when she shrieks after examining me. After some debate about how best to dislodge the engorged tick from my head—cover it in

Vaseline to suffocate it? Burn it? Pull it out with tweezers?—she decides to bring a lit match to my head and hope my hair doesn't catch on fire.

Mom grabs a box of matches from the top shelf of a kitchen cabinet and throws it on the paint-stained table like the box itself is hot to the touch, both of us staring fearfully at the red-and-white Diamond logo. With shaking hands, Mom reaches for the box, gingerly picks up a match, and swiftly runs it over the striking surface before bringing the hot flame dangerously close to me. Feeling the flame approach, my natural survival instincts kick in and I jump off the chair and run, screeching, into the living room, convinced that my entire head will be set ablaze. This goes on for several more failed attempts, until Mom finally gives up and yanks out the engorged tick with tweezers.

1989
After the tick bite, my childhood health vacillates between periods of being relatively normal and exhibiting random inexplicable symptoms that change as quickly as adolescent best friends. I wake up one morning in fourth grade with my fingers curled into claws, my hands burning as though set on fire and the ache in my knuckles unbearable. The pain lasts for weeks before Mom reluctantly schedules an appointment for me, certain I'm just being overdramatic.

My first positive test for Lyme disease was three years earlier, and the two-week course of penicillin my pediatrician prescribed at that time did nothing to assuage my symptoms or ward off the army of Lyme bacteria setting up camp in my young body. Now I test positive for Lyme disease again and begin another ineffective round of penicillin. The discovery of Lyme disease is still in its preliminary stages at this point, and there's little research or understanding about the long-term consequences or best course of treatment.

I take the small opaque brown bottle of penicillin to school with me and swallow the tiny pill with my carton of milk at lunchtime. One of the lunch monitors notices and harshly reprimands me for bringing medication to school without notifying the nurse's office. I'm mortified that she yelled at me in front of the entire fourth-grade class and immediately begin to associate sickness with doing something wrong. I sheepishly walk through the lunchroom with hundreds of eyes staring and fingers pointing, my blushing face cherry red with humiliation.

The penicillin helps incrementally—either that or I just get used to living with the dull throbbing pain throughout my joints. The memory of my teacher's raised voice is so traumatic that I stop mentioning any further ailments to anyone, including my parents, for fear that I'm wrong and will get yelled at. This is the start of my being accustomed to living in a constant state of discomfort, my new normal.

My body takes its sweet time before turning on me completely. Persistent stomachaches, cramping, and digestive issues begin to consistently plague me, forcing me to lie down on the couch in agonizing pain after dinner most nights, too uncomfortable to finish my meal yet famished with hunger an hour later. Mom is convinced there's a perforation in my stomach lining, and so I choke down a warm chalky barium solution in her radiology clinic, terrified of the eerie dim lighting and sounds of the X-ray machines. Mom steps behind the lead-lined walls and tells me to stay still, then she watches and critiques as the tech scans my stomach looking for tears, blockages, or tumors.

The scan reveals nothing—my insides are the picture of health, according to the grainy black-and-white pictures. This leads to one conclusion: I must be faking. My issues are chalked up to being a picky eater, and I suffer through dinners by pushing peas around my plate and hiding food in my pockets before excusing myself several times to the bathroom to flush chicken and tenderloin down the toilet. I am so tired all the time that I sleep through the loud buzz of two alarm clocks each morning while the annoying pitch travels through the house rousing every other family member before someone finally shakes me awake.

Although he doesn't tell me until later in life, Dad is convinced I have an eating disorder. A late bloomer and one of the smallest in my class, I am a dwarf among giants, enviously eyeing the budding breasts of my friends while my chest stays flat and size-zero clothes hang loosely off my pale skeletal frame.

An eating disorder wouldn't have been all that surprising as Mom dies a few years later when I am only 16 years old. I am certainly not equipped to grieve such an enormous loss, and I come to rely on unhealthy vices to cope. But an eating disorder is not the root cause of my failing health.

Vast quantities of Busch Light and late-night pizza deliveries in college accelerate my body's decline. I consume bottles of Pepto-Bismol and Tums like my GPA depends on it. I literally shit my pants one day while running to the dorm bathroom. Stuffing my underwear into the tampon disposal bin, I hobble back to my room in wet, foul bell-bottom jeans and tell my roommate I need a shower to freshen up and—come to think of it—should probably do a load of laundry as well.

The fatigue gets worse while I get better at ignoring it, and my shrill alarm clock now wakes up every freshman on the seventh floor except me. I reluctantly go to the university health clinic and am diagnosed with late-stage mono, the overworked nurse practitioner telling me that there's nothing to do except wait for the exhaustion to pass, that I'll be feeling better in no time. The tiredness never eases up, and I am perpetually fatigued.

Convinced I contracted a parasite during a trip to Mexico before the start of my junior year of college, I leave the university clinic with a brown paper bag and a stool specimen collector. I shove it as far into my backpack as it will go lest someone catch a glimpse of it. Once again, the test results show that I am healthy as a horse, the doctor attributing the gastrointestinal distress to anxiety.

Weight begins melting off my slender frame in my early twenties as a gray pallor takes over my fair complexion. My stomach issues worsen, now coupled with shortness of breath. I seek out a gastroenterologist, whose advice is to eat more fiber to help the constant bloating and cramping. Metamucil and cardboard-tasting wafers are not the answer. An endoscopy and colonoscopy, while providing a crystal-clear view inside of me, provide no further answers to my health woes. The doctor runs a full blood panel, and his nurse calls me in a panic the next day, leaving several messages on my answering machine before I answer.

"Sarah, I've been trying to reach you all day. We need you to come in immediately."

"Sorry—I was snowboarding and just got home. What do you mean? What's wrong?"

"*Snowboarding?* How did you possibly have the energy for that? That's too dangerous right now! You are severely anemic, and I emphasize *severely*. If you fell and hurt yourself or started bleeding, you could die. We need you here as soon as possible for a blood transfusion."

I spend the next few weeks receiving transfusions to raise my red blood cell count up to a stable level. Once these normalize, I require regular iron infusions for months. During my first iron infusion, I go into anaphylactic shock and swell up like an overinflated balloon, the breath in my chest cut off until the nurse pushes epinephrine through the IV catheter in my arm to counteract the reaction.

Specialists from all different areas—hematology, oncology, gastroenterology, neurology—are puzzled. After each appointment, I'm left with more questions than answers. The oncologist subtly throws out the L word. Not Lyme—leukemia. My symptoms prompted her to consider cancer, and she orders a bone marrow biopsy for further testing.

It must be the anesthesiologist's first day out of medical school because I feel every inch of the large needle digging into the back side of my lower-left hip bone, a lightning bolt of pain shooting through my iliac crest and down my leg as the doctor aspirates bone marrow out. My screams of pain make my stepmother cry as she steps out of the room to avoid fainting. The doctor tells me he didn't get a large enough sample on the first try and that he will have to go back in, just one more poke and it will all be over.

I beg him not to, pleading with him like a prisoner of war. "No, no, no, I will do anything—just please don't stick that needle in me again."

Burning and writhing in agony as they hold me down, my anguished cries are muffled into the flat antiseptic-smelling pillow as sweat soaks my navy and baby-blue velour jumpsuit. When it's finally over, my face is streaked with tears as I close my eyes in relief.

I do not, in fact, have leukemia or any other form of cancer. The official diagnosis after many professionals review my chart is celiac disease, an autoimmune disorder where the small intestine is hypersensitive to gluten, leading to difficulty digesting food and absorbing nutrients. I am so happy to finally have an answer, and I feel so relieved believing that all my health issues will be solved just by eliminating gluten from my diet.

I have forgotten about my childhood diagnoses of Lyme disease, and I don't mention them anywhere on my health history forms, blissfully unaware that Lyme disease affects the digestive tract and can mimic other disorders.

These health trials are only preparing me for what is to come years later.

CHAPTER 3

In Your Head

JANUARY 2017 – AUGUST 2017

The initial warning signs of chronic illness are all too easy to ignore. They creep in slowly, gradually, incongruent and irrelevant to one another, until one day you wake up and realize you are unable to function the same way you did the day prior.

Stopped at a red light one blustery January morning while driving to the gym for my usual grueling workout, dark wormlike eye floaters begin swimming lazily across my eyes, distorting and blurring my vision as though I'm looking through a screen. My head feels fuzzy, dusted with cobwebs that have accumulated overnight. There is a menacing sense of something being off; unable to identify what it is, I shake my head vigorously to rid myself of this sensation but experience no relief. Instead of turning around and driving home to rest, I respond the way many of us do when our body is trying to communicate with us. I look the other way.

My mentality has always been "all or nothing." There's no room for the murkiness of gray areas, and I enjoy living in the definitiveness of black and white. I blame these new odd sensations on motherhood, convince myself that the past few years of sleep deprivation have finally caught up with me, shrug them off, and put them quietly in the back recesses of my mind. I am determined to lose the last stubborn pregnancy pounds and will not let something as trivial as eye floaters or brain fog deter my workout routine.

Nolan is twelve years old, Everly is four, and Addy is two and a half. Becoming a full-time mother while also working part-time from home requires a delicate balancing act, ensuring a proper allotment of time each day to my career, motherhood, spousal, and household duties. The girls accompany me to the gym every morning and spend two hours playing with their friends at Kids Club while I work out to the point of sheer exhaustion with the other gym moms. Noticing that my workouts are becoming increasingly difficult, I decrease the intensity and add in relaxing sauna sessions and whirlpool time, which do nothing other than make me feel more tired.

After a challenging TRX class, I stare at myself in the mirror and feel a deep sense of foreboding. My arms are heavy, my body is filled with lead, and my shoes are made of boulders. Crushing fatigue quickly slinks into my daily life and makes it necessary to nap every afternoon while snuggling with the girls on the couch as they watch a movie, leaving me with a great deal of guilt for using a screen as a babysitter.

Every day brings another new, unwelcome symptom, all of which seem completely independent and unrelated to each other. The eye floaters I experienced several months ago are now taking over my vision completely, the fatigue so debilitating I am unable to work out and must cancel my gym membership, isolating me from friends and social interactions. An increase in moodiness and lack of libido strains our marriage, and Dan and I fight more frequently over petty issues.

Severe brain fog consumes me, making it difficult to focus on basic rudimentary conversations. I frequently lose my train of thought mid-sentence. Chronic sinus infections stalk me for months, and I cycle on and off antibiotics every few weeks for some relief. My joints ache. The index finger of my right hand is so swollen and painful when I wake up one morning that I'm convinced it broke in my sleep. I use popsicle sticks and duct tape as a makeshift splint. I become sensitive to scents and fragrances and am repulsed by the smell of our laundry detergent and hand soaps. I exchange all our hygiene and cleaning supplies for organic, all-natural products.

I dread bedtime because even though I am exhausted, my nights are filled with restless legs, agitated sleep, and night sweats that leave me shivering in a pool of cold dampness. I rise each morning with purple under-eye circles that get darker each day and eye puffiness resembling that of a contender in a boxing match. Compulsive behaviors insidiously weave their way into my daily life and cause anxiety, fear, and irrationality. Vertigo strikes at the most inopportune of times. Shortness of breath and heart palpitations stop me in my tracks, forcing me to focus on a strong inhalation of oxygen into my lungs. Reading my Kindle one evening, the words jump around on the page as if dancing to their own musical number.

My hair starts falling out, slowly at first and then intensifying. I dread taking a shower and watching handfuls of long strands swirl lazily down the drain, sucked into the slippery abyss of pipes never to return. As vain as it sounds, this is the final straw that makes me acknowledge my new bleak reality.

I schedule an appointment with my endocrinologist, Dr. K, with whom I have a long-standing relationship due to a 2007 diagnosis of Hashimoto's disease, an autoimmune disorder that causes hypothyroidism. She orders the customary thyroid bloodwork to check my levels. When the results come in, she tells me I am the epitome of the health. She surely must have mistaken my results with those of a different patient, but no, everything looks good and well within the range of normal. Dr. K's recommendation is to get more rest, perhaps talk to a therapist to deal with the challenges of motherhood and raising young children.

Rage surges through me. I feel a strong urge to scream and yell in her face that *"Something is wrong with me!"* Thinking better of it, I compose myself and remind her of all the recent symptoms that have plagued me and beg her to do more testing. She eventually placates me. I'm sure she senses my frustration and probably just wants me out of her office. She orders a full workup including a basic chemistry panel, cortisol, adrenocorticotropic hormone, estradiol 17 beta, follicle-stimulating hormone, luteinizing hormone, automated differential DL/CL, CBC and differential, iron, and vitamin D. Once again, my test results are considered within normal range, and she has no further answers for me. I feel in my core that something dangerous is happening inside of me, but I don't know where to turn for help.

My health continues deteriorating rapidly, but I attempt to ignore it and maintain life as usual since all my lab work reveals nothing is wrong. The days become interminable, yet I trudge miserably onward. I take the initiative and change my diet. I create awful green concoctions that look terrible and taste even worse, clumpy fibrous drinks with celery strands that get stuck in my teeth. There is no noticeable difference after drinking them for a month, leaving me defeated and discouraged.

I turn to alcohol to hide from my fear. I know I am destroying and self-sabotaging my already fragile body. I feel drunk after just a few sips of wine and fail to experience the momentary escape into oblivion I so desperately crave. I question my sanity, whether I am developing hypochondriac tendencies. I wonder if everything is all in my head as the symptoms show no discernable pattern that can connect the dots to a definitive diagnosis or course of treatment. I am as lost as a metaphor.

I have the picture-perfect life on the outside. A handsome, successful husband, three beautiful children, and the ability to work from home on a part-time basis while maintaining our household and raising our kids. We travel frequently due to Dan's career obligations, and friends are often envious of our tropical retreats. I become quite adept at projecting an image that reflects extraordinarily little of my true reality. I do not consider myself sick yet and will hide behind the mask of a healthy person for as long as possible.

Dan's yearly Managing Director conference is at The Atlantis resort in the Bahamas. Waking up before the sun, we pile three sleepy kids and several overstuffed suitcases into the truck and drive to O'Hare airport for an early direct flight to the Bahamas. Addy, who has a history of getting carsick, does not disappoint. Shortly before arriving at O'Hare, she throws up all over her favorite cupcake blanket, which I throw directly into a garbage can in the parking garage, prompting an ear-splitting screaming tantrum that lasts several minutes. My patience is already worn thin, my anxiety is through the roof, and I am unsure how I'm going to make it through this long travel day.

After checking our bags and making it through the extensive security line, Dan and I order mimosas. We drink them as we walk briskly to our gate and welcome the sweet thrill of champagne into our bloodstream. The small amount of alcohol makes me feel disoriented and dizzy, and I gladly nod off for a few hours once the plane leaves the runway and the kids are settled in with their coloring books and iPads.

The sprawling Bahamian property is lush and beautiful. "Who has it better than we do?" is a regular phrase among our colleagues, but the frequency with which we jokingly repeat this saying belies my true darkness. We spend the week living in a real-life aquarium, ride inner tubes underneath a shark-filled lagoon, walk below stingrays flapping their bodies languidly against the reinforced walls of the tank, and marvel at the magnificent creatures that call The Atlantis their home.

I maintain my carefully crafted façade of health and participate in company activities and meals, utilizing any free time to lie down by the pool and watch the kids splash around in the shallow end. While lounging at the pool one afternoon, an unsettling sense of paranoia disarms me, and I begin trembling fiercely, adrenaline coursing through my veins and putting me on high alert. I scan my surroundings, certain someone is going to kidnap my children or me. I am moments away from running to a lifeguard for help when Dan notices my shaking and proceeds to calm me down slowly and bring me back to reality. This is my first true anxiety attack, which deeply unnerves and disconcerts me. Dan brings me a piña colada and I frantically gulp it down, desperate for the rum to kick in and take the edge off.

The Atlantis boasts a lengthy rope bridge, an iconic walkway over the shark-filled Predator Lagoon. The kids are adamant that we walk across, so I plod along after them. I close my eyes constantly behind my sunglasses because I can barely keep them open in the heat. My lungs are not able to get enough air, and the shortness of breath is exhausting. Not wanting to disappoint my family, I fake a giant smile and traipse across the unsteady rope bridge. Vertigo immediately sets in, and my line of sight becomes smaller, ending with a pinprick of light as though I am standing in the middle of a long, dark tunnel. I stop dead in my tracks, holding onto the scratchy twine sides of the bridge for dear life with knuckles white from the intensity of my grip. The people behind us are clearly annoyed as they wait for me to move forward. My entire focus is on breathing, and I eventually put one foot in front of the other and make it to the other side as strangers huff and brush past me rudely. I reveal none of this to Dan or my father and stepmother, Candy, who are vacationing with us.

Later that evening, my folks watch the kids while Dan and I attend a company dinner. After half a cocktail, I am so lightheaded and unsteady on my feet that I excuse myself early, skip dinner entirely, and retreat to the safety of our room. The children, sun kissed and exhausted from today's activities, are half asleep when I return, and Dad and Candy tiptoe down the hall to their room a few doors away. Listening to Addy's quiet murmurs of "I puked...I puked...I puked on my cupcake blankie," I tell myself I am merely jet-lagged and that traveling with children is exhausting for anyone, desperately pretending that nothing is wrong when everything is wrong.

CHAPTER 4

Runaway Train

SEPTEMBER 2017 – DECEMBER 2017

The fall and winter of 2017 are some of the most physically debilitating days of my life and bring no relief to my failing body and mind. I am not ready to fully admit defeat yet, but I can no longer deny that something is gravely wrong. I fake everything and pretend to be who and what I once was—healthy, vibrant, confident, well. The veil of a healthy person that I have been trying to wear is growing too small and will not fit for much longer.

I cling to the small glimpses of my former self that occasionally resurface, which provide refreshing breaks and fleeting moments of lightness and levity in my marriage, a welcome respite from the usual tension that tethers us loosely together. These moments are short-lived as the constant reminders of sickness grow larger by the day. I stop getting my period and can barely see through the screen of eye floaters that relentlessly cloud my vision. I am living in a stranger's body. Paranoia and self-loathing multiply exponentially, bone-crushing fatigue takes over, and the only thing that sounds good is sleep. Following a conversation is excruciating, and I float along in a dreamlike state, not quite here and not quite on the other side either.

My existence is becoming intolerable. I struggle to stay afloat, keep my marriage intact, and raise our children. Everly attends the morning session of 4K, and although her school is a one-minute walk directly across the street, I can barely make the brief trek to her classroom without getting winded and dizzy. The 600 feet from our driveway to the front doors of the school may as well be 600 miles. I stare out the dining-room windows and think that there is no way I can walk that far. Yet I do. Of course, I do. As a mother I will do anything for my children. I reluctantly force myself out of bed when I would much rather stay nestled beneath the warm caress of the soft gray duvet and ignore the reality of my life. I will rise from the dead every morning, climb the unscalable mountain, and walk into the raging inferno for my children. So, I do. Day after more unbearable day. Addy and I trudge home after dropping Everly off each morning, and I immediately put a movie on for her so I can sleep on the couch for the few precious hours until pickup.

The girls begin to notice I am not my usual self. Even though they are young, they can sense the tension that permeates and lingers throughout our house, and their sticky hands cling to me more than usual. Their neediness is a nuisance and an additional burden that I cannot be bothered with, and I often sneak away to the confines of our bedroom to hide under the covers. Everly always finds me minutes after I disappear, her hazel eyes watering and chin quivering, not fully comprehending why Mommy needs to rest so much, devastated that I do not spend as much time playing with her as I used to. Seeing her pudgy little cheeks streaked with tears is a knife to my heart, a painful reminder of what a terrible mother I have become.

Demons are lurking everywhere—the reflection in the mirror, the judgmental stares from strangers at the grocery store when I do venture out, the disappointment on Dan's face when I reject his advances once again. Convinced everyone is out to get me, paranoid and suspicious of all those who cross my path, I turn inward into the dark hole of desperation that I can only describe as severe depression. I am constantly wondering when I will reach the black abyss of the bottom. Anger and rage encompass me. I am humiliated for getting sick and not being strong enough to fight off whatever has taken hold of me. I feel a scarlet letter of disease branded onto my entire being. I become unrecognizable, a shell of my former self. I retreat from friends and family, from Dan, from my children.

The inexplicable shame that accompanies the loss of my health shakes me to the core. I lose any remaining scraps of self-confidence. I feel ugly, dull, gray. I question why Dan would still want to be married to a wife who has nothing left to offer, who is boring and worthless, who is apathetic and not interested in any form of intimacy or affection anymore. I am my own worst critic. I beat myself to a pulp and begin to hate myself with a self-deprecating vengeance. I unapologetically lash out at Dan and the kids for the most trivial of things, desperately trying to find an outlet for the fire-hot anger bubbling through my veins right below the surface, a volcano waiting to erupt.

My heart is black, extinguished of all joy and happiness. I am undeserving of their love and affection and feel the need to punish myself for the horrible human being I have become. I do not deserve to be happy anymore because I am sick without any proof of illness.

Losing faith in finding a quick fix for my ailments, I search for alternative ways of healing outside of the traditional Western medicine box and read numerous holistic healing books, determined to find answers that might help me. I stumble upon functional medicine, a concept that focuses on identifying and addressing the root cause of disease rather than just the symptoms, a theory that is foreign to me. I Google providers near me and come up with a limited list of results, deciding on the one whose office is closest to home.

My first appointment with a functional medicine practitioner, Dr. Michele, is in December 2017. The intake forms alone take 30 minutes to complete and are more comprehensive than any other medical paperwork I have filled out in my life—pregnancies and childbirth included. The clinic runs a litany of bloodwork prior to me seeing the doctor, after which the lab tech escorts me into an examination room.

I wait for several minutes until Dr. Michele bursts through the door full of enthusiasm, her arms waving wildly and a frantic energy emanating from her. Tall with a somewhat masculine build offset by her dark pixie haircut and porcelain freckled skin, she is assertive, direct, and no-nonsense. Instead of a typical welcome and formal introduction, she accusatorily screeches, "Why have you been on Prilosec for fourteen years?!"

Stunned into submission and feeling like a child who's done something wrong, I fumble my words. "Uh, well, you see, I, ah, I had really horrible acid reflux when I was younger, and my gastroenterologist told me to take Prilosec, so I listened to him?"

I hope that turning my explanation into a question and transferring the onus onto my prior doctor will put me in Dr. Michele's good graces, but it does not seem to do the trick as she stands over me, her wild eyes boring into me until I finally look away.

"Um, I can stop taking it?"

"*Yes!* I cannot believe you have been on it for so long. Hasn't any other doctor mentioned this to you? You're only supposed to be on it for two weeks at a time."

Shaking my head, I say, "No, I don't think any of my other doctors gave my medical history or intake forms more than a cursory glance. They all seem to think this is fine."

"Well, they are wrong. Your gut has been destroyed by it, and it's going to take a great amount of work to rebalance your digestive system. Contrary to popular belief, acid reflux is not the presence of too much stomach acid but rather a *lack* of stomach acid whereby you cannot properly digest your food, which then comes back up your esophagus and results in inflammation. You need to stop taking this immediately."

"OK, but what am I supposed to do then for the burning pain?" I am terrified of stopping Prilosec because of the fire-breathing dragon that resides within that will rear its scorching head upon missing even one dose, but I'm committed to getting to the root cause of my failing health.

"I recommend natural digestive enzymes, which may take a while to work but are effective. Also, your lab results indicate many of your hormone levels are off, as well as vitamin and brain chemicals. All of this leads me to believe that, in addition to your autoimmune disorders of celiac disease and thyroid issues, there is another chronic disease at play. I'm not sure what it is yet, but I'm going to start you on a strict supplement regimen."

I see the words spill out of her mouth, hear the intricate medical jargon with my own ears, but she sounds like the teacher in Charlie Brown: "Wah wah wah." Nodding along to the quick cadence of her voice, I frantically scribble in my notebook so I can look up the definitions of the words she throws at me—estrone, GABA, glutamate, cortisol—and try to make sense of them later.

As the receptionist hands me a heavy bag of supplements and the lengthy post-appointment paperwork, I gasp when I see that the total payment due nears four figures. I am instructed to take a total of 49 pills each day, some on an empty stomach, some with food, some 30 minutes away from food, some only during the week and not on weekends, some only at bedtime. I create a spreadsheet with dosage and timing instructions and follow it religiously, ensuring I take all pills as directed. I do not feel any different after two weeks, but I stay optimistic and look forward to the holidays, hoping that Santa will fill my stocking with good health this year.

We celebrate Christmas Eve at the home of my brother, Matt, and sister-in-law, Sierra, but first we stop at a random church on the way for an early service. During the service, I get misty-eyed and choked up when the lights are dimmed and candles are lit for the traditional chorus of "Silent Night." I'm overwhelmed by the beauty of the hymn and the parishioners quietly singing along in the flickering soft glow of the white candles.

We arrive at Matt and Sierra's with brightly wrapped packages adorned with curlicue ribbons and tinsel bows, bottles of wine, white elephant gifts, and appetizers. Santa Tracker is on the television screen and all the children anxiously peer out the large bay windows every few minutes in search of Rudolph's red nose, certain they can see the outline of a sleigh in the distance. I briefly mention my health issues and supplements to my family, slyly pop smelly pills into my mouth, and downplay the true severity of my failing health. Until I have an official diagnosis, there is not much sense in thinking about what-ifs or going down blind rabbit holes worrying about what may or may not happen.

Matt pops two bottles of champagne, and after a boisterous toast and clinking of glasses, we dig into the charcuterie board replete with olives, cornichons, prosciutto, Genoa salmi, soppressata, cured sausage, Brie, cheddar, Manchego, Gouda, and Parmesan. I pair these with a few gluten-free crackers, and several minutes later I am in the worst agony. My throat begins closing in on itself and the fire-breathing dragon is ready to burst through my skin. I run to the foyer and grab my purse, pop open the bottle of Zypan, and swallow digestive enzyme after enzyme, hoping for some relief, which does not come. The entire bottle is not enough to dull the raging inferno in my throat.

My heart races and my face turns beet red as heat rapidly rises through my body. I hear the laughter of the children and the lively conversation of the adults from the kitchen and quietly slink off to the playroom to lie down on the faded couch. Feeling alone and scared, I contemplate calling 911 for help, certain that a heart attack is imminent. My stepmother comes to find me and not wanting to alarm my family and reveal how terribly sick I truly am, I tell her I'm just tired and need to rest for a while. I feel too embarrassed to admit that I am dying.

CHAPTER 5

Steal My Sunshine

JANUARY 2018 – APRIL 2018

    The dreary gray days blur seamlessly into one another, the passage of time marked solely by the ticking of the clock and turning of the calendar pages. The lack of sunlight does nothing to help my mood or outlook, and I increase my vitamin D intake—which produces no noticeable difference. I research seasonal affective disorder, try on a self-diagnosis of this and try to squeeze myself into that box. No matter how much I scrunch, suck it in, and lie to myself, the diagnosis just will not fit, and finally I give up shoving a round peg into a square hole. Six weeks have passed since my initial visit with Dr. Michele, and although I don't feel any better, I'm still hopeful that the next sunrise will find me healthy and whole again.

    Questioning the validity of my symptoms makes me flip-flop like a fish out of water, wavering between utter devastation at my declining health and bouts of hope when my symptoms subside for a few hours. Anxiety skulks in like an unwelcome guest, evasive and undetected while I'm securely cocooned in my home but making its presence known as soon as I step outside the safe confines of my four walls. A trip to the gas station or grocery store leads to a sharp increase in heart rate, followed by shortness of breath and perspiration soaking through my shirt and staining the armpits.

    Happiness and joy turn into strangers. Emotions I once knew so well are now unrecognizable. The many blessings surrounding me have become burdens, and I struggle to find any sense of meaning in life. The beautiful smiles of my children are the only things that keep me going, forcing me to find the good in each day and focus on anything positive, no matter how small it may seem. Did I wake up this morning? Yes! Was I able to get out of bed and walk of my own volition to the bathroom and brush my teeth? Yes! Am I still able to provide and care for my children? Kind of! The gratitude is fleeting as other emotions and thoughts rush in. Doubt, fear, worry, discouragement, self-hatred, and thoughts of death quickly take over and consume me. I am caught up in the agony of being me. I unintentionally sabotage and destroy relationships, never stopping to think about how my sickness is affecting others or how they are feeling. Illness is slowly becoming my new identity, rendering it impossible to see anything outside of my own pain and suffering.

Dan is struggling with this mystery illness that has taken over our lives but does not know how to support me. I cringe when he touches me and reject all his advances, the tiny fissures in our marriage now widening into a large chasm. Talking is exhausting, and our conversations become very one-sided, Dan asking all the difficult questions and doing the hard work to save our marriage while being met with one-word monotone responses from me. He sits alone in a tub full of bubbles with his single champagne flute while I nap in a fitful sleep on the couch. Frustrated and alone, he reaches out to our realtor, Gary, with whom he has begun to develop a friendship.

They meet a few days later at the Gingerbread House, a quaint cozy café in a historic farmhouse with chickens running around the large wraparound porch. After ordering two black coffees and getting settled at a small table with tiny metal chairs, their conversation begins with them catching up on each other's business and seeing how they can assist one another professionally. Gary talks about the state of the real estate market and Dan discusses the ever-changing nuances of the financial services industry. The typical pleasantries and business talk quickly turn to what is happening in their personal lives.

Dan shares the details of the rapid decline of my health: the inexplicable symptoms slowly sucking the life force out of me, the numerous doctors who cannot figure out what is wrong, the shift in my personality and energy. Gary nods along, vehemently shaking his head with understanding, and excitedly tells Dan about the decade-long quest he and his wife, MK, went on when she experienced symptoms like mine. After ten long years of misdiagnoses, numerous cross-country trips to see a myriad of specialists, and thousands upon thousands of dollars later, they finally found a doctor who understood what was happening and why.

This conversation between Dan and Gary changes the trajectory of my healing path and, I strongly believe, saves my life.

After hearing about their talk, I immediately call Gary for more information, feeling the tiniest glimmer of hope that someone else might actually understand what I am going through. We meet a few days later at Panera, along with MK, and sit outside in the sun as we sip our dark-roast coffee. I describe the deterioration of my health, the puzzling symptoms that come and go, the brain fog, fatigue, vertigo, heart palpitations, shortness of breath, the countless signs that something is wrong with me. Gary and MK punctuate the nodding of their heads with murmurs of recognition—mmm-hmms and yeses after everything I say, buoying my hope that I am not alone.

MK shares her story and describes what she went through, an experience very similar to mine albeit with a longer timeframe. She tells me of the great relief she felt when Dr. Jay Davidson came into her life. Dr. Jay nearly lost his wife to Lyme disease twice, and through trial and error, he finally learned what was needed to save her life. He took everything he learned and turned it into a protocol. He wrote and published a book, *5 Steps to Restoring Health Protocol*, to share his knowledge with others struggling from chronic Lyme disease. He was unlike any doctor MK had seen prior, and he immediately thought she had Lyme disease. She had several bouts of testing, including the ELISA test, the first step in a two-tiered approach to diagnosing Lyme disease. This test detects antibodies produced by the body's immune system in response to the bacteria that causes Lyme disease. The ELISA is falsely negative half of the time, so it's not very effective or accurate. The second test is the Western blot, which is more specific than the ELISA test. The results of her tests were undeniable: she had late-stage chronic Lyme disease.

The initial relief MK felt at having an official diagnosis was tempered by what would be required to regain and restore her health. Dr. Jay's methods did not include antibiotics, prescriptions, IVs, hospital procedures, or mainstream medical techniques, and the cost of working with him was not covered by insurance or any healthcare plan. He used all-natural methods, food as medicine, and was strongly rooted in a functional approach to healing. There was no quick fix or magic pill, just the promise of remission with time, effort, and patience. It took years, but MK was eventually able to fully recover her health by following his protocol. The conviction and belief both she and Gary have is palpable, and I feel something tug at me to investigate Dr. Jay further, to keep this in the back of my mind as I am still hopeful that Dr. Michele will be able to help.

My next appointment with Dr. Michele is a few weeks later, and I tell her I may have Lyme disease. She scoffs at my remark. She's flippant and dismissive, and I immediately feel embarrassed for advocating for myself. The mere mention of Lyme disease changes her entire persona, almost as though she is scared to broach the topic. She mentions the inaccuracies of testing and how results are not truly an indicator of whether a patient has Lyme. Called "the great imitator," Lyme disease can mimic other diseases because it has symptoms that are similar to many other illnesses. A voice inside keeps nudging me and I am adamant that she tests me. She finally concedes and orders the lab work. My blood is drawn, and the waiting game begins.

Several days pass with no phone call or update from her office. I am restless and impatient, nervous I have Lyme and even more concerned I don't. I call her office and am told my results are indeed in and she will call me back later. She does not call me back later, and over the next five days I call her office several times a day, only to be told she will get back to me when she has time. I am so angry that I physically start shaking every time I pick up the phone attempting to reach her. I consider driving to the office and demanding she speak with me. My personality and reactions are not mine anymore, and I cannot trust what I might do or say when I get to her office. I'm so enraged that she holds the fate of my health in her hands and is too preoccupied to even call me with an update.

When the call from Dr. Michele finally comes, I pick up before the first ring finishes, blurting out an annoyed huff of a "hello." My blood is boiling at her lack of attentiveness and concern for my well-being, yet I try to remain calm because I want answers. There should be a simple answer but with anything Lyme related, there is no such thing as simple. Dr. Michele restates what she told me prior regarding the ineffectiveness and lack of accuracy with testing, the chance of positive negatives and negative positives. She tiptoes around my actual results and refuses to give me a definitive answer.

I listen to her drone on as long as I can before asking her point-blank in frustration, "Do I have Lyme disease? Yes, or no?"

Sighing in annoyance, she mumbles, "Well, it's kind of like being pregnant. You can't be just a little bit pregnant."

Rolling my eyes, I clarify: "So I do in fact have Lyme disease."

Her silence on the other end is deafening, as though saying the words out loud will make her sick by association. If she will not officially diagnose me, then I will do it myself. I. Have. Lyme. Disease. I thank her for her time and realize she does not have the necessary breadth of experience to address my illness. I request a copy of my chart and that all labs be emailed to me and know I will never see her again.

CHAPTER 6

Down with the Sickness

APRIL 2018 - JUNE 2018

The disappointment from working with Dr. Michele is blunted by the excitement of investigating Dr. Jay. My health (or lack thereof) becomes my obsession. It preoccupies my every waking minute, each new lead a potential magic wand of healing. It is easy to get lost in the multiple rabbit holes promising a quick fix, and I spend countless hours scouring Dr. Jay's website, digging up any information and watching every single video of him on the internet. Devouring his book in one sitting, I pray the answers will jump off the page at me and that just by reading it, osmosis will set in, the power of the words transferring into my body and making me well. When this does not miraculously happen, I call his team to determine if working together may be a good fit, only to discover he is not accepting new patients. But, they tell me, his colleague is, and I schedule a—very expensive—call with Dr. Nick for a week later.

Before the initial 90-minute Skype consultation, I complete an extensive health history questionnaire even more detailed and in-depth than the one at Dr. Michele's office. Nontraditional questions cover a wide array of topics, including everything from dietary intake of pork products and bottom-dwelling sea creatures to use of aerosol hairspray, to the presence of silver fillings (mercury) in my teeth, to any recollection of being bit by a tick. I have no idea how all these things can possibly be related, but I try to keep an open mind.

Several days later, Dan and I sit side by side in Dan's office so we can both see Dr. Nick on the screen. I am nervous, apprehensive, and a bit giddy all at once, knowing he has taken the time to review not only the lengthy questionnaire but also the pages of prior doctor records and lab results. I'm hopeful he can provide some answers. After brief introductions and a general synopsis of the decline in my health, the first question he asks is whether my symptoms get worse during the full moon. My heart sinks, and Dan and I squeeze each other's hand under the table, as we both think, "What the hell did we just pay all this money to this quack for?" Too polite to end the call after seven minutes, I tell him I do not pay much attention to the moon cycle, so I have no idea if it results in worsening of symptoms.

Our conversation continues for the next hour and a half like this, Dr. Nick asking questions out of left field and me responding with a lot of "I don't know" and "I've never thought about that." I tell him about the dietary changes I've already made, the green concoctions I blend that taste like dirt and the strict gluten-free diet I adhere to. He says that if my diet were the only thing wrong, I would be doing much better than I currently am.

Deciding halfway through the call he legitimately knows what he is talking about, I unequivocally know he can help me and I want to work with him. He thinks I am certainly an eligible candidate for this program and will be able to reclaim my health by working with him; his team will be in touch soon to coordinate further details.

We hang up, and I release a flood of tears onto Dan's shoulder. I know this is going to be difficult but I don't fully understand the enormity of what I just signed up for. It will take months for me to realize just how far-reaching the effects of Lyme disease have been on my body. I question the strength and determination it will take to get through this next year and doubt my commitment to healing, especially knowing how long it may take. Dan reminds me he will be right there alongside me, supportive and encouraging every step of the way, and that he's on board with whatever I need to do.

The email from Dr. Nick's assistant, Allie, greets me the following morning with a comprehensive list of instructions and expectations for working together. This health-coaching program is not covered or reimbursed by any form of insurance, and I must pay out of pocket for everything. Lyme disease is a very lonely and expensive world, but I am a dead woman walking, a prisoner in my own body, so I am willing to pay anything to feel even the slightest bit better. I complete the formal coaching paperwork and mail it to their office, along with a check greater than five months of mortgage payments. The wheels are in motion, and there is no turning back now. The program consists of nine one-hour virtual appointments every thirty days, each month building upon the prior with protocol instructions based on how my body reacts. My first official coaching call is one week later.

The call goes slightly over the allotted one-hour time limit, and I am left with pages of scrawled notes and a huge list of new supplements to order. Lyme disease sufferers never just have Lyme. There are usually several coinfections accompanying it—mean tickborne diseases that like to play, naughty bullies on the playground pushing and shoving all the nice little kids down. The initial symptoms of Lyme disease are fever, headache, possible rash, and fatigue, all ailments of the common cold or flu. Because of this, sufferers are left vulnerable and exposed to the later and more crippling stages of Lyme disease when it moves into the joints, heart, and nervous system.

This next month will consist of dramatic diet changes. Following a strict gluten-free diet for over 15 years due to the celiac disease diagnosis in my early twenties forced me to make dietary modifications, but the changes Dr. Nick recommends up the ante to an entirely new level. He tells me to cut out dairy, sugar, soy, all grains, most fruits (berries in moderation, cherries, grapefruit, avocado, and Granny Smith apples are acceptable), and nonorganic vegetables. If any food has more than one ingredient, I should not be consuming it. I scan the labels and multi-ingredient items in the pantry—why on earth is titanium dioxide in our food and banned in Europe, and how many people are oblivious to this?—and throw over half of the food into the garbage.

Grabbing my reusable grocery bags, I head to the store and stock up on organic vegetables, green apples, sweet potatoes, lentils, beans, raw coconut oil, flaxseeds, hemp seeds, chia seeds, Primal Kitchen condiments, raw nuts (not peanuts though, as they are bio toxic), and quinoa (it is a seed, not a grain, and does not turn to sugar in your body). I substitute my beloved Wisconsin cow cheese for sheep-milk alternatives to maintain some sense of normalcy. Once home, I unpack and stare at the bland bounty in front of me, Hippocrates' words echoing in my mind: "Let food be thy medicine and medicine be thy food." I plaster my Advanced Eating Plan sheets to the cabinet, the words blurring as tears fill my eyes.

The second focal point this month is getting my body to drain properly and create better flow throughout the lymphatic system, which plays a crucial role in removing toxins. For those of us with compromised immune systems, improper drainage results in toxins being recycled throughout the body, leading to decreased immune function and illness. To assist with opening my drainage pathways, I begin taking tinctures, homeopathic drops, and pills of all shapes and sizes. I purchase two very large pill boxes to organize the chaos of my eight-times-per-day supplement schedule. Thirty minutes before each meal, I take digestive enzymes and two tablespoons of raw unfiltered apple cider vinegar with water (my gag reflex is strong even with my nose plugged). I also invest in a portable infrared sauna and a set of dry brushes, both of which are meant to open drainage pathways and stimulate the removal of toxins.

But the best way to help my body detox? Coffee enemas. Not comprehending the words that come out of Dr. Nick's mouth, I ask him to repeat himself and sure enough, he says clear as a bell, "You will do coffee enemas two to three times every week."

"Sorry, come again?"

Dr. Nick does not sugarcoat anything. He is very direct and to the point. "Coffee enemas. They're not as bad as they sound. They stimulate bile flow, toxin removal, and the production of glutathione. You can buy a stainless-steel kit on Amazon. Make sure the coffee is organic and light roast. I'll email you full instructions on how to perform this."

Laughing uncomfortably and realizing this is not a joke, I think about shoving a hose up my ass and letting my colon enjoy a nice cup of light roast. When I commit to doing something, I dive in headfirst and put all my energy into it. There is no middle ground. I am either in or out, go big or go home. Working with Dr. Nick does not mean that I can pick and choose the easy parts and ignore the difficult ones. For this to work, I must be all in, and so I purchase an enema kit on Amazon and wait for it to arrive the next day.

Our second coaching call is one month later, in early June. There are no noticeable changes in my symptoms yet. Dr. Nick reminds me to be patient and that natural healing takes time. The first month was all about changing what goes into my body and opening the drainage pathways. Month two is the introduction to the start of a parasite cleanse. Yes, parasites. I quickly realize Dr. Nick is bringing things to light I previously had no idea even existed. Parasites are for third-world countries, for children who grow up in squalor and do not have access to clean water, for those living in filth, among fleas and scabies, where there are no professional medical resources. Parasites are not for me, I thought. I was so naïve.

Dr. Nick explains that everyone has parasites, but most people can maintain a symbiotic relationship with the organisms living inside them. For those of us with compromised immune systems, however, parasites tend to take over, laying eggs and multiplying at an alarming rate, wreaking havoc on the human body and weakening their host. Ignorantly believing parasites are microscopic bugs, invisible to the naked eye, I tell Dr. Nick I can handle this—it will not be an issue. Let's get these nasty little buggers out of me as quickly as possible.

In addition to the slew of daily pills from the month prior, I add several antiparasitic supplements. I begin slowly and then increase the dosage as my body gets accustomed to them. The spreadsheet of all the supplements, dosage, and timing instructions to keep things straight is now spilling over onto two pages.

Dr. Nick tells me I will probably be a little uncomfortable to start. The first two weeks of taking the antiparasitics leave me with a rumbling stomach and slight gastrointestinal distress. Week three (during the full moon), I receive an email from Dr. Nick instructing me to double my dosage for the next ten days. New and unsettling sensations course throughout my body within 24 hours of the increase. Intense abdominal cramping appears out of nowhere, and it feels like there are tiny suction cups on the interior of my stomach, tickling me from the inside as they undulate and pulsate throughout the day. Things move underneath my skin. A tiny slippery something has made its way into the back of my head and is swimming lazily around up there, invading my body, which seems to be no longer mine but belongs instead to a foreign alien creature.

I increase the frequency of my infrared sauna usage, binding supplements, and coffee enemas to help alleviate and minimize these terrifying sensations. The morning after the particularly disruptive night of the full moon, I get the kids off to school and rush home to do a coffee enema. I let the light roast organic coffee cool just enough in the French press to not burn my asshole or innards, then I insert the coconut oil-covered tube into my anus and slowly release the lever, letting warm fluid flow inside me. Lying on the cream-colored bathmat with a faded pink towel over it in case my bowels and large intestines do not cooperate, I stare at the white walls and oak trim of the bathroom floor and wonder how I possibly got here, with a hose of coffee up my ass, a supplement schedule that surpasses that of a 90-year-old in a nursing home, and a diet where my dessert consists of a green apple. I close my eyes and sigh, then a minute later I feel the strongest urge to run to the toilet even though the liquid has not been held inside of me for the recommended amount of time. Nothing could have prepared me for what happens next.

There are several three-foot-long slimy rope worms floating in the toilet amid the tan hue of the organic coffee I just expelled. Three. Feet. Long. Several of them. I stand there, naked, horrified, shocked, disgusted, yet morbidly fascinated all at the same time. Should I take pictures of them? Scoop them out and dissect them? Send them somewhere for testing? They are not moving and are clearly dead, and a wave of relief passes over me as I realize the supplements worked and I should start to feel better any day now. Before I can overthink anything, I flush the toilet and away they go.

One of the perks of working with Dr. Nick is that I always have access to him. I can reach out to him on his cell phone in between scheduled appointments if there is an urgent need. This seems urgent, so I call Dr. Nick, after taking a long, soapy shower, to tell him what I saw and that all the parasites are out of me.

He chuckles. "Oh, Sarah. This is just the beginning."

"I'm sorry, come again?" I realize this is becoming my typical response to him. "What do you mean, this is just the beginning?" My excitement at getting rid of the nauseating worms deflates like a week-old birthday balloon.

"I'm glad to hear you got a few out, but there are likely hundreds of those inside of you with how sick you are. They lay eggs constantly and are very difficult to kill. Parasites are most active during the full-moon cycle, which is why I told you to increase your dosage so you have the best chance of killing some of them."

"Sooommmmmmme of them?" There is a slight delay as my brain attempts to register what he just said. "So how long until they are all gone?"

"I can't say for certain, but you will be on a parasite cleanse for at least the next twelve months."

"Twelve *months*?!" I shriek.

"At least. Stay positive. It's incredibly encouraging that you are already eliminating these from your body in just a few weeks. I am here to help you, and I know you can do this."

We hang up, and the weight of his words sinks in slowly. Reality and disbelief intertwine and mingle together in one giant fucked-up cocktail. How on earth did these massive worms get into my body and how was I so ignorantly unaware they were living inside of me? Was it from drinking tainted water while traveling to Mexico? Sipping directly from a crystal-clear stream in the high mountains of Telluride years ago? Did I eat worms in fruits or vegetables and then they made my body their home? There will never be a definitive answer to this question, and at this point it's irrelevant. The only thing that matters now is getting them out as quickly as possible. Now I understand why Dr. Nick asked if my symptoms got worse during the full moon. My resolve sets in, and I am more committed than ever to taking back control of my body and making it my own again. I am completely unprepared for what lies ahead of me.

CHAPTER 7

So Low

JULY 2018

The next few weeks are a blur of cramping, bloating, worms, headaches, tears, f-bombs, and severe distress. The physical symptoms are horrific as the parasites happily await the strong diabolical energy of this moon cycle to lay their eggs and procreate inside of me, using my blood and intestines for shelter and nourishment. Their slimy slippery bodies swim frantically through me in anticipation of the full moon, and I feel them stronger than usual this month. I see them pulsating in my right knee, their snakelike bodies squirming and wriggling like worms pushing to the surface after a heavy rainfall.

The emotional symptoms are even worse. Signs of the body breaking are pain and weakness; signs of the mind breaking are underlying fear and neurotic thoughts. My mind becomes a persistent record on repeat, the off button nowhere to be found. I am plagued with disturbing, morbid thoughts and nightmares, the stuff of which horror movies and serial killer documentaries are made.

I dream that my deceased brother is being run through a meat grinder, his blood and guts pushed out through those tiny little holes like sausage. Waking up in a cold damp sweat, scared and unable to make sense of what I just experienced in my mind's eye, that image is forever seared into my brain. Escape is impossible. I try to think about baby bunnies and rainbows, but the sinister thoughts overwhelm all else. Murder, death, carnage, and gore encompass my days, and I am repulsed by the thoughts in my head. I'm reluctant and unwilling to admit to anyone what is happening. A song by Self from my teenage emo angst years plays nonstop in my head: "I'm so low, that I wish I was dead, with a knife in my chest, and a bullet through my head. I'm so low that I wish I was dead. Must I go on?"

My soul is clawing its way out of this human body, scratching, scraping, itching to be released. Reluctantly mustering up the strength to get out of bed after that terrifying nightmare, I force myself into the shower. The scalding water cascades over my aching body as deep, painful, soul-wrenching sobs pour out of me. I cry over the hesitant acceptance of the loss of my health, the lack of answers, the crumbling state of my marriage and the vast expanse of distance that illness has created between us. I cry for the strong sense of self-hatred and loathing that is there every time I look in the mirror, and I cry for losing myself and the person I once was. I completely understand how people who are battling this choose to end their life; it seems a preferable alternative to the daily torture of living with this disease.

I call Dr. Nick in a panic. I can barely articulate words through the hyperventilating gasps that escape my lips. I plead with him incoherently for answers to what is happening.

I whimper, "My entire body is breaking. I'm neurotic, depressed, compulsive, too anxious to leave the house. Everything hurts. I just want to die. I'm being fractured in half and I'm so scared. What is wrong with me?"

Dr. Nick, even-keeled as always, responds, "Sarah, parasite and toxin die-off can result in not only physical symptoms, but emotional symptoms as well. The parasites are doing everything they can to stop you from killing them, and they are going to make you as uncomfortable as possible. Your body has been through a lot these past few months and still has a very long way to go. Now is a time to be gentle with yourself and rest as much as possible."

"I don't think I can do this," I say. "It's all too much for me to handle. There's so much pain everywhere—in my body, in my mind. I don't even want to move." I am not yet aware of the connection between the body and the mind, that you cannot heal one without the other, and I still think of them as two separate, distinct pieces.

Fearing I am on the edge of a nervous breakdown, Dr. Nick takes a deep inhalation and exhales it forcefully. "Sarah, I need you to breathe right now. Just breathe. In...and out...in...and out. That's better. Keep breathing with me."

My heart rate slows down and the chatter in my mind eases ever so slightly.

He continues. "I think it would be prudent for you to talk to someone who is better equipped to handle the emotional aspect of chronic illness, as this is not my area of expertise. I want you to reach out to Islena Faircrest. She has helped several patients who are suffering from chronic Lyme disease, and I think she may be able to help you as well."

I nod in silent agony, thank Dr. Nick, and hang up. I rest my weary head on my crossed arms on the kitchen counter and slump my shoulders in defeated surrender. I remain there for several minutes or several hours—time is meaningless right now—before eventually pulling myself up and reaching for the phone again. I do a quick Google search on Islena, which reveals her background as a holistic therapist and trauma-informed life coach with expertise in early childhood and family development. Trusting Dr. Nick and his advice, I hesitantly call her and am greeted by a soft, melodic voice on the other end.

After speaking with her for a few minutes, I envision her being the kind of person who takes daily walks to hug her favorite trees and undoubtedly dances outside naked under the light of a full harvest moon. Regardless of my juvenile initial judgment, something about her voice has an immediate calming effect and my intuition is pulling me toward her. Deciding I have nothing to lose by scheduling one formal coaching session with her, we pencil in an appointment together for two days later.

Islena is fifteen minutes late for our first call. I am annoyed and strongly debate cancelling our session before it even starts, but upon hearing her voice again, my irritation instantly disappears. She wastes no time and dives right in. She describes seven different areas of our lives: spiritual, financial, family, social, physical, mental, and vocational. At different times in our lives, we experience pain in different areas. She allows me a few minutes to write down and think about each one and then asks, "Which one—or more—do you think is out of balance right now?"

"Ha. Where do you want me to begin?" I cynically reply. There is pain in most of these areas, but the one standing out the most, which is also the most difficult for me to openly admit, is the mental area.

Islena perceives my hesitancy to answer her question and ignores my poor use of sarcasm to deflect. "Good. We have a starting point. Let's think about a time in your life when you felt the need to be strong. Take a few minutes to reflect and let me know what pops up for you."

"I don't need to think about it—that's an easy one. My mother died when I was sixteen years old, and being the oldest of four kids, most of the responsibility fell on my shoulders."

My throat involuntarily constricts, and a lump begins to well up there, making it difficult to speak any further. These are familiar sensations that arise whenever I talk about Mom, and the others soon follow: the red-hot flushing in my cheeks, formation of sweat beads on my forehead, adrenaline coursing through my veins as if a tiger were chasing me. I do everything in my power to think of something else, to hold back the well of tears threatening to spill over because I do not want to cry in front of a virtual stranger less than ten minutes into our conversation. I cannot possibly let my guard down and show any sign of weakness.

"Ahhh...I see."

The intonation of her voice makes me feel like she can see the physical reaction I am having to the mere mention of Mom's death, as though she feels my pain and sympathizes with the hurt 16-year-old still living within me. This uncanny ability of hers feels simultaneously like an invasion of my deepest secrets as well as a relief that someone else is finally seeing a sliver of the real me for the first time. I feel exposed and on display. Her demeanor and intuitiveness are both welcoming and intimidating.

She continues. "I am so sorry you had to deal with this, but we need to explore this further as it is a trauma experience and a clear source of pain. Sarah, I want you to get curious and explain how you feel when you think about your mom. Tell me where in your body you feel a sensation and then describe it. What does it look like—is it round, flat, square? What color is it? What does it taste like? Smell like? What does it feel like—is it sharp, smooth, jagged, prickly?"

Our conversation is quickly escalating into unpleasant territory. I bristle with discomfort like a hissing tabby cat arching her back at a stray dog and plead, "Do I really have to do this? This is making me extremely uncomfortable. I just want to know how I can get better."

Islena purrs back in a delicate, tranquil tone. "I can tell. And, yes, this is important. Close your eyes and tell me what you see."

I huff sharply in disgust and belligerently squeeze my eyelids together. "Fine. I feel something in my throat. It is round, bright red, a hot pulsating fireball. I feel something black and jagged in my chest. It is sharp and will cut me with even the slightest touch."

Islena makes the smallest chink in my armor after only 30 minutes, and I cannot hold back the tears this time.

"Good, Sarah. This is really, really good. I want you to place your hand over your heart now and drop into your sixteen-year-old self. Think about what you were wearing, who your friends were, what you did for fun. Tell me about that—use specifics."

I physically recoil at her words and despise thinking about this time, yet I do as she asks. "I was probably ditching class and smoking Marlboro Reds in my trusty beige-and-white oversized GMC Jimmy by myself. After Mom died, most of my friends distanced themselves from me and I didn't have anyone to eat lunch with in the cafeteria. When I wasn't ditching class, I would eat by myself in the library, pretending to read encyclopedias for a nonexistent research project. I was wearing Airwalk sneakers, oversized JNCO jeans, and a snowboarding T-shirt. I used to play on the volleyball and soccer teams, but I dropped out after Mom died."

"Wow. That paints a great picture. Tell me more about the deterioration of your friendships."

"Once Mom died, a cord was severed between my classmates and me. I was so different from the other students. I was alone, trapped on Motherless Island while everyone else was still nestled comfortably on the Island of Two Living Parents. I felt cheated, lost, scared, trapped, isolated, and so very sad. I was completely unprepared for the great burden that was thrown in my lap of stepping up and taking care of my three younger siblings. My world just collapsed around me, and I had no other choice but to push through. I still had to wake up every morning and take care of my family—"

"Very much a parallel to what you are currently doing right now with your own health crisis," Islena interjects.

I miss the insight of her comment, see no correlation between how Mom's death could be related to my illness now. I just want her to tell me what to do to get better. I keep going.

"We all put on an act and pretended that everything was OK in the wake of Mom's death. This was our coping mechanism and the only way we knew how to deal with the situation. Dad had time to prepare in the months leading up to it. I always held out hope that she would miraculously get better one day. Surely there was a doctor smart enough to fix her, to cure the cancer that had spread to every part of her body, right? She was only forty-nine years old and had four children to raise. How dare God take her away from the family who so desperately needed her? It was not fair. I'm frightened that my destiny is aligned with Mom's and my children will be motherless soon."

I am shocked that I am opening up so freely to someone I barely know.

"How did your father respond and react to losing his wife?"

"Dad did the best he could. He presented structure for us, kept the family functioning, provided love, stability, and we never wanted for anything financially. But we didn't talk about feelings. We went to one family counseling session but none of us were willing or ready to talk. I went to school the day after Mom died and pretended I was unfazed by her death."

Islena jumps in as if she has just found the last missing puzzle piece. "Ahhh. This is all coming together now. Your psyche was not able to process the traumatic event that just occurred. The safest thing for you to do at that time was to follow your father's lead and set an example for your three younger siblings. The five of you were all clinging desperately to your own life jackets to just stay afloat and not drown. It was not good or bad, right or wrong. It just was. It was what you all had to do to survive."

I furiously scribble in my journal as she continues. "These circumstances created a survivor in you. You needed to keep the peace, and you likely held yourself to impossible standards trying to keep your family intact. Most teenagers are not equipped to run their family unit. You rose to the challenge because it was necessary, and you succeeded. The missing piece is this came with a huge price tag: you did not navigate your feelings and you bypassed the grieving process to ensure your family's survival. This response is not relevant anymore, and it's been irrelevant for quite some time. You just haven't been aware of this until now."

Sitting in stunned silence with tears running down my face, I question how she can possibly know all of this. I marvel at her uncanny ability to read me.

"Your own illness is forcing you to grieve your mother's death properly. Ignoring feelings does not make them go away. You need to forgive your sixteen-year-old self for avoiding the grief and for not understanding how necessary it was for healing. You need to thank her for keeping your family afloat. You did nothing wrong."

"I should have been there for my siblings more, for my sister, who was only twelve. I was so focused on my own pain that I neglected theirs and—"

"No, you did enough. You are experiencing emotional anguish, coupled with your physical pain, because you are not equipped with the resources to properly navigate your feelings. This is what we are going to work on together. I want you to write this down: 'I, Sarah, am going to successfully learn the tools to navigate my feelings and emotions, identify them and where they came from, *feel them*, allow them to move through me, and neutralize them. I will use this experience to not fear my emotions anymore.'"

My homework before our next session is to digest this call, journal about my feelings, and email my thoughts to Islena. Our call has gone well over the allotted one-hour time limit, bordering on almost two hours. Exhausted and spent, I collapse on the dining room floor with my eyes closed and try to comprehend what just happened. Our conversation was awkward, unpleasant, and well beyond the confines of my comfort zone. It is exactly what I need.

CHAPTER 8

Red, Red Wine

AUGUST 2018

Life doesn't stop because I am sick. Dan turns 40 in a few weeks, and his dream for this milestone birthday is to celebrate with friends and family in one of our favorite places, Napa Valley. We honeymooned there and have many fond memories of the beautiful landscape filled with tapestries of vineyards, multicolored hot air balloons, majestic sunsets dipping below rows of freshly planted vines, and the air ripe with the smell of crushed grapes. I want everything to be exactly right for him. Months earlier, I spent a great deal of time booking winery tours for us and a large group of friends, reserving a block of hotel rooms, hiring a Sprinter van to drive us around, and making the perfect dinner reservations.

I have yet to disclose the full extent of my illness to family and friends. They know my health has been subpar for some time now, but it's difficult to explain my condition when I don't fully understand it yet myself. I am sick but I am not. I am here but I am there. I want to die but I want to live. I am still able to participate in most activities and show up for life, unlike many who are lying comatose in a hospital room incoherent and unable to perform the daily activities of living. Never one to seek the sympathy of others or throw myself a pity party (I did go to school the day after Mom died, after all), I prefer to keep problems to myself, to internalize them so as not to burden others.

It is very early on in my healing protocol, and although I am not in denial that I am sick anymore, I still hold a great deal of defiance about my plight. I very much want to live a normal life while navigating chronic illness. Dan will only turn 40 once, and I refuse to miss this trip after putting in all the time and effort of planning it, no matter how bad I feel. I put my best foot forward and don the mask I've been wearing in public lately. I gear myself up to be a healthy person for the next four days. But the mind can only do so much before the body inevitably breaks down.

The warm California air kisses our cheeks as we cruise with the top off of our four-door cherry-red Jeep Wrangler rental and drive to the heart of wine country. The wind whips through my thin hair and tangles my wispy strands into a knotted mess. We sing horribly off-key to "Getting Drunk on a Plane" as we pass by the large "Welcome to this world famous wine growing region" sign. We slow down as we drive through downtown Yountville, and I take in the small-town charm of Washington Street, the main drag lined with tasting rooms, shops, art galleries, and boutique hotels. Considered the culinary capital of Napa Valley, Yountville is home to one of America's top Michelin-starred restaurants, The French Laundry, which is just a stone's throw away from the antique inn where we are staying.

The concierge of Maison Fleurie warmly greets our group with a wide smile and freshly baked cookies as we check in. The history of the legendary oldest hotel in Napa Valley is evident throughout the property as decorative knickknacks brought over from France complement the beauty of the lush rose gardens surrounding the pool area.

The morning of Dan's fortieth, I arise early, bloated from the long day of travel and eating salty airport snacks and exhausted from a restless night of sleep. I put on a tacky "OMG HE'S 40" T-shirt and decorate our oversized king suite with cheap birthday decorations. After a quick breakfast, our driver meets us in the gravel parking lot, where we take pictures in the haze of the early-morning light and playfully tease one of our friends who looks rather queasy from the night before, fiercely clutching his Gatorade bottle like a life raft. We boisterously board the large Sprinter van and after a quick stop at the Oakville Grocery to pick up our preordered boxed lunches for later, we begin the day's festivities by popping several bottles of champagne on the way to the first winery, glasses clinking and loud party music blaring through the speakers.

I turn the music down several octaves and shush everyone like a librarian to disruptive students and ask them to be quiet while I give a speech prepared the hour prior. I express my gratitude to each person there, thank them for joining us for such a special day, for their friendship, for the joy they bring into our life, and for being some of our closest friends whom I consider family. Words get stuck in my throat as emotions overcome and wash over me like a wave. My chin quivers and my voice wavers, very atypical to my usual calm and cool personality, but I quickly dismiss this, brush it aside, laugh it off. I feel like a fraud, a liar, a cheat, because this group of people, who are supposed to know me best, still have no idea who I truly am or what I am going through. My desire to clue them in to the secret I have been hiding is overpowered by the immense amount of embarrassment I feel for being so different from them, for tiptoeing quietly into the kingdom of the sick while they are still happily in the kingdom of the well. I take a sip of my mimosa and wait for the alcohol to hit my bloodstream and dull my thoughts and emotions.

I participate in wine tastings like I have in trips past; however, this time I pour more wine into the spit bucket than I consume. The tannins of the Pinot, the sweet honeysuckle aftertaste of the sauvignon blanc, the deep, jammy purples of the Cabernet, and the effervescent bubbles of the champagne that wink flirtatiously from their flute, all beckon me to come drink them like an old friend. Although I love the taste, I cannot tolerate alcohol like I used to, and I'm tipsy after two tastings. I drink bottles of water back on the van and munch on packages of Paleo Puffs and grain-free snacks that I packed in my suitcase. We feast on our boxed lunches at an estate overlooking evenly spaced rows of vines and rolling hills. The dazzling bright color of the sapphire pool lies in stark contrast to the yellow, green, and auburn hues of the natural terrain. I take in the view and close my eyes. I soak in the rays of the sun and the tickle of grass between my toes, the perfection of this moment, and feel a single tear roll slowly down my cheek.

It is a magical day and the laughter on our limo bus is plentiful, but by the time we get back to the hotel, I cannot act anymore. My brain wants to stay and have fun with our friends, cannonball into the pool, laugh at stupid jokes, drink more champagne, live recklessly in the moment. My body does not agree, however, and starts shutting down. I tremble violently, and I'm sure I will faint in the next minute, so I excuse myself and retreat to the safety of our room to lie down and rest. Dan follows several minutes later, ready for his—ahem—*real* birthday present. And although I try my best to be engaged and excited about our intimate alone time, I pass out, physically unable to keep my body or brain functioning and online.

Two hours later Dan is gently shaking me awake and whispering in my ear, asking if I want to shower and get dressed to go out for the evening. I manage to shake my head no, crushed by the fact that I can't join the group for my husband's birthday dinner. He kisses me gently on the forehead and quietly shuts the door on his way out. I stare at the ceiling and notice a tiny spider in the corner. I wonder if it's weaving a web of lies as large as the one I have woven around my health. I lie there for hours, listening to the faint sounds of drunken laughter trickle in through the window, alone with the aftermath and repercussions of straying from my usual strict diet.

I crawl to the bathroom and throw up the contents of my stomach, my body eagerly ridding itself of all the toxins I so foolishly ingested. I throw up until there is nothing left, spit long strings of putrid yellow bile into the toilet, and swear I will never touch a drop of alcohol again. I will start listening to my body more, will let it run the show instead of my brain. I am tethered to my pre-sickness life, and I don't know how to cut the cord, how to be a sick person. I don't know how to remove my mask yet. Once my stomach stops roiling and the rancid taste in my mouth has lessened to a manageable degree by several swipes of the toothbrush and gargles of mouthwash, I shuffle to the bedroom and collapse onto the soft pillowtop mattress.

Early-morning sunshine filters in through the white cheesecloth curtains, as Dan forgot to close the louvered shutters when he got home last night. My heavy-lidded eyes squint open at the brightness that envelops our room and quickly squeeze shut a moment later as I perform a mental scan of my body. I want to curl up in a ball and die. My body is frozen to the bed and refuses to move. This is not a hangover; it feels like something sinister is eating me from the inside. *What have I done? What is happening to me?* I lie there with a racing heart and frantic eyes as Dan snores softly next to me. Ten minutes pass as feeling slowly returns to my achy limbs and joints, allowing me to gently wiggle my toes and fingers. I sluggishly reach for my phone on the nightstand. I call Dr. Nick in a panic, and he picks up on the third ring.

"Hi, Dr. Nick. It's Sarah. I'm in Napa, and I am freaking out. I woke up this morning with numbness in my limbs and heart palpitations. I have some feeling in my fingers and toes now, but should I go to urgent care?"

"Woah...slow down. Walk me through the past three days—your diet, physical activity, sleep."

"As you know, it's Dan's birthday, so we flew to California two days ago. I've been trying to eat healthy, but I've been indulging a bit and had some wine. Sleep hasn't been great the past few nights at our hotel."

"You're having a Lyme flare-up and you're experiencing worsening of symptoms. Flare-ups are triggered by everything you just mentioned—alcohol, processed foods and sugars, poor-quality sleep. Muscle stiffness, numbness or tingling in hands and feet, and general body pain are common symptoms during a flare-up."

"What's the fastest way to get rid of this?"

"You already know that answer, Sarah. Follow your diet, stay away from alcohol, and get some rest. Your body is always talking—you just need to listen to it. Take it easy today, perhaps get a massage or take a nap."

I thank him profusely as we hang up. I know his advice is accurate but will not be heeded on this last day of our trip. Understanding the importance of saying no and actually doing it are two different things.

I turn on the shower, watch my reflection soften as the mirror fogs up with steam, relish the feel of the hot water that soothes my aching body, and linger in the warmth until the water turns cold. I swipe my hand across the hazy mirror, pull myself together, and remind my distorted reflection of who I am: the tour guide of this trip, the one in charge, the cruise director leading the electric slide on the lido deck. I had planned another fun day of wine tasting—chardonnay, rosé, pinot noir, Moscato, champagne, merlot, something to please everyone in our group—so I courageously plaster on the fake smile that I hide all my suffering behind and open the door, ready to face another day of bad decisions and poor choices. *It is only one more day*, I whisper to myself. *I can do this. I'll deal with the consequences when I get home.* The show must go on, and I do not want to disappoint anyone. In the meantime, I'm oblivious to the fact that I'm disappointing myself.

CHAPTER 9

Head Above Water

SEPTEMBER 2018

I pay a very high price over the next three weeks for our trip to Napa, including lying restlessly in bed for ten hours each night as new symptoms attack from every angle. I question the intelligence of my decision to go to wine country in my condition, berate myself for not staying home and resting, then dismiss that thought with the saying "Life's too short, tomorrow is never promised."

One of Dan's cousins is getting married in Chicago four weeks later, a joyous occasion that we would not miss for the world. Because Dan attended a work conference in New Orleans the three days prior to the wedding, I pick him up from the Milwaukee airport on our way to Chicago. Pulling up to the curb in Big Momma, my behemoth SUV, with the kids and luggage secured snugly in the back, I stare at my husband standing there, looking handsome as ever with his dark sunglasses on and chomping on a piece of gum like a valley girl, both signs of a late evening.

I put the hazard lights on and hop out to give him a hug and a kiss. I smell the stale scent of booze that lingers on his breath. His words are raspy and his eyes ruddy and bloodshot from the long night before. I am instantly triggered and furious. Hatred and jealousy emanate from every pore as anger bubbles over and scalds me like a boiling pot of hot water. He went out with a group of coworkers, enjoyed some adult beverages, and stayed up well past midnight, something that has occurred in the past and has never been an issue for me before. He works hard to provide for our family and deserves to blow off steam. I have always been secure in our marriage, knowing we have a rock-solid foundation built on trust and mutual respect, never once questioning his intentions or his love for me. My irritation directed at him today is unjustified, my emotional outburst and irrationality surprising both of us.

We spend the rest of our car ride mostly in silence, his attempts at conversation punctuated with my one-word responses and exasperated huffs. I'm still seething when we check in to the hotel and get settled. Dan, clearly sensing my sour mood, gently pulls me aside and quietly asks what is wrong.

"Nothing. I'm fine."

That evening, which also happens to be the 14th birthday of our oldest child, Nolan, we celebrate the rehearsal dinner with a large family gathering at a Brazilian steakhouse. Gauchos cut enormous slabs of meat as guests flip their coasters from green to red, red to green, stoplights missing their cautionary yellow color. I stick to the salad bar, hoping that flare-ups and symptoms will subside with a cleaner diet. I munch on asparagus, fresh vegetables, plantains, and gluten-free yucca balls while everyone else piles their plates high with parmesan-crusted pork, steak, bacon-wrapped chicken, dry-aged tomahawks, lamb chops, and wagyu.

Laughter and heat rise with the consumption of meat and wine, and the initially inviting room becomes stuffy and suffocating. Panic and anxiety pop up without warning, emerging like a terrifying jack-in-the-box and make my blood run cold. I survey the room as my anger lurks nearby, hidden in plain sight between the laughter and merriment of the crowd. I want to lash out at the cheerfulness surrounding me as inexplicable wrath explodes inside me like fireworks. My palms turn clammy and sweaty. The napkin on my lap is damp with moisture, and I tell Dan that we need to leave *now*. We say rushed goodbyes, hop in a cab, and retire early to our hotel room, my heart rate and anxiety only returning to normal once I hear the click of the door latch and see the security chain firmly in place. We sing Happy Birthday to Nolan and ooh and ahh as he unwraps his coveted Lego set, say our prayers, and go to sleep. I am so angry at Dan that I toss and turn all night, listening to him snoring loudly beside me.

The cheerful sun is in sharp contrast to my gloomy mood. Last night's fitful and restless sleep leaves me with dark circles under my eyes and a grayish-blue pallor to my complexion. I pinch my cheeks in a sorry attempt to get some color in them and tell myself to suck it up, there is nothing wrong with me, stop being a little bitch and get over myself. Flinging open the bathroom door with a frenzied smile, I help Everly and Addy into their adorable mother-of-pearl cream flower girl dresses, curl their hair into ringlets, and ensure their barrettes are positioned just so. I throw on my own dress and apply a light dusting of makeup, a layer of camouflage to get me through the day. After a quick breakfast in the lobby, we board a trolley with the rest of the bridal party to the church. Addy and I sit a row ahead of Dan and Everly, so I don't have to talk to my husband, and Nolan sits by himself in the third row. We smile brightly for all the selfies on the ride there, the sunshine and warm fall air disguising my darkness inside.

The ornate Catholic church is breathtaking, decorated simply yet beautifully in traditional fall colors and flowers. The burnt-orange roses, majestic black-eyed beauty and sunrise Calla lilies, warm pink succulents, and bright golden-yellow sunflowers give subtle pops of color to the otherwise stark white and gold interior. The traditional ceremony is a tearjerker. Dan and I beam with pride when Nolan reads from First Corinthians and gasp as the Matron of Honor almost faints mid-ceremony from the heat. Our daughters are the cutest flower girls. The ruby-colored rose petals they throw flutter lazily down the red-carpet aisle like slow helicopter tree pods taking their sweet time before hitting the ground. I am simultaneously flooded with love for my children and this budding new marriage and miserable at the deep-rooted hatred and anger that envelops me.

By the time the reception rolls around, I am holding myself together by a fraying thread, barely containing the flood of tears in the dam of my eyes. I flit anxiously from here to there, a bee sampling nectar from a field of flowers, never staying in one place long enough to have more than a perfunctory conversation with extended family members. My paranoia is heightened—I am certain they are talking behind my back, questioning Dan about my odd mood and distinct change in behavior. After dinner, I sit solemnly at a back table and try to remain invisible. I sulk and glare at the terrible dance moves of the tipsy revelers. Dan's aunt notices me sitting by myself and walks over and asks if something is wrong. Am I OK? Do I want to talk?

Her words break me, and the tears flow as I crossly tell her that of course I am fine, nothing is wrong, I'm just tired. My venom is now pointed in her direction. I'm angry at her, angry at the whole room, angry at the world, an animal backed into a corner baring her teeth, ready to fight everyone even though they are only trying to help. I want to run out of that room, away from the dance floor, the forced laughter, the music, the drunken speeches, and clinking of glasses. I want to run away from my life.

I push myself up from the table with more force than necessary, jostling the half-empty glasses of cheap wine and barely eaten pieces of wedding cake. I scan the room for Dan and the kids and stalk toward Dan as fast as my three-inch heels will let me. I tell him it's getting late; the girls need to go to bed, and I need to rest. He and Nolan can stay and dance some more. He protests and I turn away from him. I grab Everly and Addy by their hands and stomp off toward the elevator, using the girls as pawns to regain some sense of control over my life and rebalance the power dynamic in my marriage. They stare up at me and whine, "Mommy, Mommy, we want to stay! We don't want to go to bed!"

The elevator doors open, and we walk in silence to our room. Their eyelids are heavy from the long day. I gently untangle their hair from their barrettes, brush out their golden locks, help them into their jammies and brush their teeth, and they are asleep on the pull-out sofa within minutes, their cherub faces the picture of innocence and perfection. I lie in the lumpy hotel bed and stare at the muted television, fire and anger pulsating red hot within me. I try to make sense of my feelings but find it difficult to see anything outside of this storm cloud of rage.

Dan and Nolan come back two hours later, and although I am still wide awake, I close my eyes and regulate my breathing, pretending to be asleep. Dan gives me a hug and a kiss as he slides into bed, and I stay stiff as a board. I know my hatred and anger are grossly displaced, yet I am unable to direct it elsewhere. I hate myself, the monster I have become. I can feel myself breaking, but I'm unable to control the fracture points. I'm angry at the weight of everything all at once and distinctly nothing.

Dan still doesn't understand the full extent of my illness or mental state, and although I love him with every fiber of my being, I hate him for this. Hate him for not being more intuitive, for not being able to read my mind. Hate him for still living his life like nothing is wrong because I feel like I can't truly live mine. Hate him for not saying no to work obligations on my behalf, for making me feel guilty if I do not want to attend events with him. I mentally and physically cannot do what I used to. I know he thinks I'm exaggerating my symptoms, and I wish I looked as bad as I felt so he would finally understand, so that *everyone* would finally understand, how miserable I truly am. I pretend, I pretend, I pretend. I pretend to love him, pretend to love myself, pretend to love our life and our family, pretend to hope that I can get better, pretend that life will ever be normal again. I am shackled to myself, to this cryptic disease, to these creatures living inside of me.

A tiny voice inside tells me I must go on, that I must go through Lyme to get through Lyme. I refuse to leave my children too early like Mom left me, and I have a bigger purpose and more to offer this world than dying before 40. Avril Lavigne wrote a beautiful song about her journey with Lyme that has been playing in the soundtrack of my mind for weeks, "Head Above Water."

A few days after the wedding, I am washing dishes at the sink and look outside at my beautiful backyard, which is in stark contrast to the gray, bleak sky. The speaker from my phone plays Avril's song on repeat, the lyrics, "God, keep my head above water," resonating and striking a chord deep within, and suddenly, the overwhelming, crushing despair and sadness literally bring me to my knees. I drop to the floor and rest my forehead on the smooth surface of the golden oak wood. My deep sobs obscure the noise of the still-running kitchen faucet, and my tears glisten in miniature pearls like drops of water on a lily pad. There is so much pain, so much desperation, I'm being pulled under by an unseen force. It would be so much easier to just let go and let it carry me away, let it sweep my body along with the current until I feel nothing. I just want to drown.

CHAPTER 10

Whiskey Lullaby

MARCH 2, 2004

The harsh rings of the telephone early in the morning become one with the dream I am in, meshing and blurring the lines between reality and the altered theta state of my brain in those precious few moments before full consciousness sets in. I ignore the first several rings before begrudgingly rolling over and picking up the cordless phone from the nightstand, irritated that I have been awoken from my slumber before my alarm clock can do its job. At 24 years old, I am working part-time during the day while attending graduate school classes at night, and a phone call this early in the morning is atypical.

Wiping the sleep from the corners of my eyes, I groggily whisper, "Hello?"

"Sarah, it's Dad." My father's voice on the other end of the line is softer than usual, muted, as though he is calling me from underwater. "I have some bad news. He shot himself. He's dead. He's gone."

"*What?* Who? Who's gone?" My voice raises several octaves.

"Mike," Dad whispers, the pain evident in his voice.

"No, no, *no, no,* this is a joke. Tell me it's not true," I shriek. I must still be dreaming, in the midst of a horrific nightmare, sure that I misheard words that can never be taken back.

"It's not a joke. He's dead."

My body is processing what is happening faster than my mind as sheer adrenaline and terror snake through my entire being, a serpentine twisting that threatens to suffocate me, making me gasp for air. Wailing incoherently and bordering on hysteria, I stumble to the top of the stairway where my knees immediately buckle and my body drops to the floor. I lie glued to the ivory speckled carpet with the phone next to me, listening to my father's breath and quiet weeping, knowing that life will never be the same. I can see the fibers of the carpet intertwining together. I focus my vision on the individual tiny strands twirling together like children with ribbons dancing around a maypole, forcing my mind elsewhere, anywhere but this moment.

Minutes pass before I hear Dad's voice again. "Sarah, are you there?"

I snap out of my trance, pull myself to a sitting position, wipe the tears from my eyes, and respond shakily, "Yes. Let me shower and get dressed. I'll call in to work and come over to your house as soon as I can."

The next few days pass by in fuzzy obscurity as more details and revelations come to light about my younger brother. I am the oldest of four, and Mike was second in our sibling lineup, followed by Matt and then the baby of our family, Julie. We are all within four years of each other, the best of friends one week and sworn enemies the next.

Mike was a wild child, a rebel who struggled with authority and had trouble learning the same way that most kids do. He was always falling behind in school, not grasping easy concepts, and being teased for having a learning disability. He made up for this with his handsome good looks and outgoing personality, and he liked to push the limits of all boundaries. He had a penchant for ladies and alcohol from a young age. The night of his death, he was drinking heavily. He called his ex-girlfriend. She heard a "click, click, click" in the background and asked what he was doing.

"I'm playing Russian roulette," he woozily slurred.

"Mike, stop it. Put the gun down. I'm coming over."

When she got there, he was noticeably drunk, and he started playing with the gun in front of her. He put the gun to his head as she watched in fear. She talked calmly, asking him once again to put the gun down.

"Nikki, don't worry. I'm lucky. Nothing bad will happen to me." He pulled the trigger, and the bullet passed through his left temple and through his brain before settling into its final resting place in the drywall behind him.

Our family deals with this the same way we dealt with Mom's death. Life goes on as usual. We make the customary funeral arrangements. My sister and I fight with each other while putting picture boards together and then sip on Bailey's at night while reminiscing through laughter and tears. There's no talk about feelings or emotions or how we're each processing this; each one of us retreats to our own private island of grief again.

While cleaning out his apartment, I stare at the bullet hole, amazed at the damage and chaos that such a tiny object inflicted. The crime scene team cleaned up the initial gore, but I can still see flecks of brain matter splattered across the wall, decorating it like the first thin flick of paint on a violent abstract Pollock painting.

The emotional turmoil of such a shocking and unexpected event makes me question everything. How can there possibly be a kind and just God who would allow this to happen, to take away two of my immediate family members? Is the purpose of our existence here on earth purely to endure pain? Was I too hard on Mike? Should I have been nicer, kinder, more understanding of his life choices and decisions? We were in the early stages of repairing a splintered relationship, our brother-sister bond having deteriorated over the years. We would hate each other with such bitterness one day and then laugh together at Dad's house the next. I should have been there to support him more in the wake of Mom's death; if I had been, then perhaps he would still be alive.

I was going to call him the night of his death to invite him to dinner for Dad's birthday celebration two days later. I remember walking out of my grad school economics exam, the smell of the crisp air that evening, the stars dim amid the light of the city, the hint of spring just around the corner. Staring at the phone in my hand, finger hovering over the green call button of my Motorola Razr, I decided I would call him the next morning. I never got the chance.

This one decision haunts me for years, the sliding glass door that shuts seconds too soon, leaving me with the hypothetical "what if" of an alternate outcome. Would my one phone call have made a difference? If I had pushed the tiny green button instead of snapping my phone closed, would he still be alive? Could I have somehow prevented his death? I blame myself, carry a burden that was not mine to shoulder, adding it to the accumulated pile of unresolved trauma already deep within my being. I bury the pain of loss for years, realizing too late that by doing so, I almost buried myself in the process.

CHAPTER 11

Spirits in My Head and They Won't Go

OCTOBER 2018

I desperately search for anything and anyone that can help me with the inescapable desire to crawl out of my skin as my body mocks me daily with its continual breakdown and failure. There is an intolerable yearning deep within my soul that cannot be satisfied—an insatiable urge for something that is indefinable and obscure, an itch that cannot be scratched. A fervent desire to say "fuck it" comes over me and I unravel. Fuck the world. Fuck my life. Fuck Lyme. Fuck it all. I just want to be, want a year away from my life to get better. But a mother can never just be, even if she is sick. There are kids to take care of, dirty dishes and laundry to do, lunches to make, bills to pay, pills to take, toys and Legos to clean up, and love to give. I cannot possibly give anymore, and I berate myself, questioning my worth as a wife, mother, and human being.

The thoughts ruminating in my mind get louder, more paranoid and delusional, so I search for help and research unorthodox treatments, everything from energy healing techniques, sound baths, reiki, and shamanic healing to crystals, chakra balancing, and psychic mediums. Psychics have always fascinated me. Although I am still working with Islena, I am convinced that a psychic will be able to provide the quick fix I desperately long for and will have the answers to heal my mental anguish. They will be able to stare directly into my eyes, the windows into my soul and deepest secrets, to tell me how to fix myself. I hastily compile a list of healers in my vicinity from a quick internet search and frantically call all the numbers. I book appointments with the first two who answer and have the earliest availability.

Two days later, I excitedly descend the steps to the basement level of a weathered corporate building, once regal and stately but now old-fashioned, the white exterior paint peeling and yellowing like aged parchment paper. I am giddy with anticipation, bursting with joy that I will walk back up the stairs with a sound mind, leaving all my emotional baggage behind. I take a seat in the windowless waiting room. The *Good Housekeeping* and *People* magazines littering the coffee table are years out of date, the harsh overhead fluorescent lights flicker and buzz for some much-needed attention, and the fake plastic plant in the corner is covered in a thick layer of dust and cobwebs.

Psychic Stacy appears out of nowhere, startling me with her sudden presence. She calmly introduces herself while guiding me to her suite down the hallway. The room is small but tastefully decorated with two couches facing each other on opposing walls and a large throw rug hugging the center of the room. Soft music plays, and an oil diffuser puffs out a citrusy cinnamon scent. I remove my shoes and apprehensively sit on the couch to my left, not sure what to expect. Stacy gets situated on the couch across from me, sitting cross-legged and closing her eyes. An uncomfortable silence grows larger as I watch her chest rise and fall. She forcefully inhales and exhales large gulps of air before her eyes explode open, her ice-blue periwinkle irises piercing through the essence of my being.

"Sarah, it's so nice to meet you and good to see you. What would you like to get out of today's session?"

My breath falters for a moment as I am oddly choked up, and she reminds me to relax and breathe. "I've been sick for months and I'm trying to find clarity into what's going on inside of me. Physical healing has been my sole focus, but I'm starting to think there may be some mental and emotional healing that needs to occur as well."

"I see. Take a deep breath. I can tell from your posture that you are uncomfortable. Uncross your arms and remove the pillow from your lap. You are using these to shield your energetic field. Focus on your breathing. Just breathe. Good. Are you willing to let me into your space, into your energy?"

I nod, and she closes her eyes again.

"I am just the messenger, telling you what I see and hear. Your aura is gray, toxic. You have an aching sense of wondering why you are even here and what your purpose is."

This hits me like a punch directly to the gut. What *is* my purpose? And why *am* I here?

"You are detoxing your liver, your entire body. There's an H. pylori infection in your stomach, something is stuck in your throat, and an autoimmune condition is going on. Your hormones are unbalanced. You just want to drink a green juice. Your neck and jaw are tight from constantly clenching and grinding your teeth. Breathe, just continue to breathe. It's OK. This is a safe space."

I do as she says, taking in a few shaky breaths.

"You wonder why your husband stays with you. You don't feel like you are enough. You feel undeserving of happiness."

I cannot hold back the tears at this statement, and they trickle down like a leaky faucet. She has articulated what I have been feeling deep inside, that I am a failure of a wife, that Dan deserves someone better, someone fun, someone healthy. I have subconsciously been questioning what he still sees in me, why he still loves me when I have nothing left to offer him, when I am a shell of who I was, a façade of a wife and a caricature of a woman.

"You are outgrowing friendships, craving alone time to discover your true self. The missing piece for you is spirituality, and you need to have it out with God, stop blaming him for taking things away from you and start seeing what he has placed in your life instead. You've spent so many years being pissed off and angry, and I can see the sadness and despair underneath your hard exterior. Your relationship with your husband will improve as you grow your spirituality, and this illness will wind up being a blessing for you. The physical battle is only one piece of the puzzle, and full recovery will only occur once you tackle the spiritual work."

"What exactly do you mean by 'the spiritual work'?"

"Only you know the answer to that. Follow your intuition. Pay attention to signs from the universe—they are all around you and are not coincidences."

The lyrics to Coldplay's "Fix You" play in the background chatter of my brain as I trudge up the stairs after our session. I am not miraculously healed as I had hoped. I mentally scroll through all the traumatic losses I have endured in my life and now, on top of all that, I've lost my health. And my marriage may be next. I feel validated in my pain, that Stacy sees what is happening not only in my body but in my mind as well, yet I'm discouraged as I don't fully understand the spiritual work I need to do.

Three days later, I pull up to a house with an overgrown yard sorely in need of a haircut; plants, vines, and weeds trail their long tendrils across the walkway like a lazy river as I apprehensively saunter up and ring the doorbell. The license plate on the minivan in the driveway reads "WITCHY," and there is a tiny broomstick dangling from the rearview mirror. I debate getting back in my car and driving away, but the door slowly creaks open and a petite woman in her sixties with salt-and-pepper hair named Les greets me. She wears the smile of a comfortable old friend, and she ushers me inside, instantly putting me at ease.

The interior of her house is cluttered, and broomstick and black cat knickknacks cover every single visible surface. The house has the potential to be on a *Hoarders* episode in another few years. The sweet, pungent scent of incense fills the room and there is soft, melodic Celtic music playing in the background. We sit at the four-person rectangular kitchen table. Dust motes are suspended in the light filtering through the clouded glass of the dusty windows like ballerinas frozen in time mid-jeté. A fat gray cat the color of cinder ash mysteriously appears in the doorway. It eyes me up and down with a cursory glance and then struts away with its swaying hips and flicking tail as if emulating a lazy model promenading down the runway.

A colorful cloth bag sits in the center of the table, and Les asks me to pick out several of the items inside. I slowly open the bag and grab three sticks with ornate carvings on them. They remind me of an art project in third grade where we used wood-burning pens to brand designs into small pieces of wood. I instantly remember the slightly sweet aroma of the hot pens on the fresh wood as fiery and strong.

I look up at Les in confusion, and she explains that these are Ogham staves—sticks carved out of twenty different native British trees, each one branded with a unique symbol representing a spiritual meaning. These sticks are a popular method of divination, similar to tarot cards. I wonder why the hell I am spending 65 dollars to look at twigs that I could have picked up from my backyard. She describes the meaning of each one as my mind wanders aimlessly, thinking about conversations from years ago that I should have handled differently, thinking about what to make for dinner, what activities the kids have the rest of this week. My eyes glaze over as I stare at her moving lips, not registering the words coming out as these sticks mean nothing to me, do not resonate with any part of my being.

She clears her throat, snaps me back to the present, and places another bag in front of me. I gingerly reach inside and feel the cool smoothness of stones. I pick out seven of varying shapes and sizes, all with intricate markings. Les informs me that these are Viking runes, stones that have either a symbol or letter on them, another divination tool. They look like something I could purchase in the arts and crafts section at Target. My mind wanders again as I do not buy into the idea that a few sticks and stones can heal my bones.

The final device in Les's spiritual toolbox is a deck of tarot cards. At this point I'm frustrated, but I play along for the last remaining minutes of our time together. She shuffles and cuts the well-worn deck, fans the cards out in front of me, and tells me to pick whichever ones I am drawn to. I glide my hand over the deck, expecting the tattered cards to speak to me, to feel a vibration calling me, for one to jump from the deck, but I feel nothing. The cards I pull focus on loss, the devil, forgiveness, and miracles. My interest perks up; now *this* I resonate with.

Les brings out a guidebook to help explain the meaning of each card, and I wonder if I am her first client, a guinea pig she is practicing on, getting taken like a cheap carnival trick. Regardless, her words ring true and give me pause. I soak in the deeper meaning and try to remain open-minded as I look down at the cards before me. I am unsure of the true meaning behind these cards, and I feel like we're both grasping at straws, but something stirs within, forcing me to pay attention even though none of this makes sense in the moment.

As our session ends and we both stand up from the small table, Les asks if I've ever called upon my spirit guides to help me.

"I'm sorry, what?"

"Spirit guides. They're always around, watching over and guiding you."

"God has been dead to me ever since he took my mother away when I was sixteen, so I don't really believe in that or any so-called spirit guides."

"It doesn't matter whether or not you believe—they're still there." Les grins knowingly, her deep gray eyes crinkling and dried pink lipstick settling into the crevices of her lips.

I thank her for her time and tell her I will give some thought to the notion of spirit guides. As I make my way to the threshold and place my hand on the doorknob, she asks me to pull one more card. I pull the Two of Swords, stare at it for a moment, and show it to Les.

She smiles. "You think you don't know the answer, but you do."

A shiver flows through me.

The mossy pavement is soft under my feet as I walk to my truck. Our session was by no means earth-shattering, and although I do not have a renewed sense of energy or a less fatigued body, I do feel the tiniest glimmer of hope. I mutter to myself, "What the heck?" then turn my face to the sky and whisper, "Spirit guides, if you are really with me, please show me a cardinal in the next week to let me know I am on the right path to healing." I have not seen a cardinal in years—they are elusive—so I feel like this is a meaningful test.

Six days pass without a cardinal sighting. I take slow walks around our block, strain my eyes looking at trees, tell myself that the bright-red breast of a robin is that of a cardinal. Doubt and skepticism weigh heavily on my heart, and the uncertainty I have that a higher power truly exists solidifies even more.

I attend a Lyme support group meeting at MK's house on day seven of not seeing a cardinal. She is passionate about helping others heal from chronic Lyme, and this is the first event she hosts. Nine of us, all in varying stages of battling this nasty disease, squeeze around her cozy kitchen table to discuss what is working for us and what we need help with, all of us hoping that someone in our motley group has an answer or can commiserate with our pain. I open my notebook, pen at the ready, and wait to hear just the right words that hold the clue to healing. As I'm sitting there, I feel someone watching me. I glance up and out the window and see the largest, brightest, reddest cardinal staring me directly in the eyes.

CHAPTER 12

Insomniac

NOVEMBER 2018

Work obligations find us in paradise again, this time at a magnificent mansion nestled away in an immaculate gated community in Cabo. I pack a larger suitcase than normal to accommodate the bags of food I must bring; my diet is so restricted now that I carry food with me wherever I go. The hosts and their private chef for the evening greet us with large smiles and even larger margaritas. I'm drunk after three sips of the sugary cocktail, and I pour the rest of mine into Dan's glass. Candles adorn every nook and cranny of the six-bedroom house, bathing the interior in a warm glow that softens all the hard edges of both the residence and those dwelling within it. The cerulean water of the infinity pool overlooks a blossoming garden filled with pink and white bougainvillea and flowers of every variety and hue; beyond that stretches an emerald-green expanse of golf course that is home to the occasional wandering cow or stray dog. I look forward to three days of rest and relaxation and to catch up on much-needed sleep.

The setting is picturesque, something out of a reality TV show, a place that only rich celebrities have access to. Still, my awe at being here is overshadowed by my desire to be at home curled up in my own bed, resting and healing. Once again, I try to play the part of a healthy person. Our colleagues ask how I am feeling, and my response is the usual lie of "I'm getting better, just a little tired." The last thing I want to do is cast a dark shadow over our fun work vacation, so I pretend to be happy, carefree, light as a feather, all while envisioning how good it would feel to lie underwater in the pool and never come up for air.

We have dinner at a local Italian restaurant our second night there. While walking to the front doors, a sudden feeling of dread takes me by surprise. My stomach roils with queasiness and agitation and my heart quickens like a runner sprinting to the finish line. Tiny stabbing sensations pinball throughout my entire body, and I latch on to Dan's arm to steady me. I tell myself that I can make it through dinner, I am safe, we will be back at the house in a few hours.

The hostess ushers us into the dimly lit main dining area and seats us at a long narrow table in the center of the restaurant. The noise of every conversation in the room attacks my hearing as tiny cymbals crash inside my eardrums. The sinister flicker of fake candles casts ominous shadows and turns each patron into an evil camp counselor holding a flashlight under their chin while telling ghost stories. While everyone is perusing the menu and our hosts graciously order appetizers and four bottles of fine wine, I frantically scan the restaurant for the nearest exit and softly murmur to Dan that I do not feel right. As plates of bruschetta, drowned octopus, meatballs, and Caesar salad arrive, I excuse myself to the bathroom and lock myself in a stall.

Shivering feverishly, I am both freezing and on fire. My body shakes uncontrollably; I am certain I will either faint, throw up, shit my pants, or die in this bathroom stall, perhaps all four. Thoughts race through my head: *Who will find me? How long until Dan comes to check on me? How will they transport my body back home?* I remain in that stall for an awkwardly long amount of time, my agitation and discomfort showing no signs of subsiding.

The bathroom attendant quietly knocks on the stall door. *"Senora, estas bien?"*

"Si, si, un momento." After what feels like an eternity, I take three deep breaths to center myself, unlock the door, stare at the stranger in the mirror as I wash my hands, and walk back to the table.

Amid concerned looks, I self-consciously sit back down and mutter to Dan, "I need to leave. *Immediately*." The look of disappointment and annoyance on his face crushes my self-worth. The two of us exit the restaurant into a waiting cab. The ride back is interminable; I am in agony, pain radiates everywhere, and my mind is assaulted by nervous system sensory overload. Once back at the house, I march down the stairs to the quiet refuge of our guest suite and immediately fall into bed, exhausted and tired, yet I find sleep just out of reach. Dan puts his swim trunks on and wordlessly walks upstairs to the infinity pool.

I develop a nasty cold once we return home, my weakened immune system lacking the resources to do anything other than keep me alive right now. It has been ten months since my last period, my body unconcerned with procreating, and although I do not miss my monthly cycle, this is just another sign of physical and biological dysfunction. My nervous system is going haywire. It's stuck in flight mode, the vagus nerve short-circuiting, sending involuntary tremors through my arms and legs with increasing regularity.

It has been months since my last full night of uninterrupted rest. I am unable to achieve any sort of restorative sleep. Instead I nod off for several minutes of fitful twilight slumber before being jolted awake by a bolt of lightning striking me. I wander the house at all hours of the night, an unsupervised toddler roaming free, and stare out the window at the pale moon that shines on me like a spotlight and illuminates all my darkness. I shake and stretch my twitching legs, lie spread-eagled on the living room floor at 3:00 a.m., and incessantly stumble down multiple rabbit holes questioning if I will ever overcome this sickness. The lack of sleep magnifies and amplifies everything—noises, thoughts, sensations, pain, paranoia. I hear my pulse in my ears, the rushing whoosh of blood through capillaries. I see my veins pulsating and throbbing with each heartbeat.

Random songs get stuck in my head for days at a time, rendering it impossible to think about anything else other than those lyrics, a record on repeat with only one melody. I hum "Rosanna" for six days straight only because it rhymes with the adaptogenic herb Schisandra I am currently taking to help improve liver function. Time simultaneously speeds up and slows down. I become a woman in a time-lapse photograph, stationary and unmoving while life goes on around me, the lights and people blurring and swirling as I stay rooted firmly in place.

The change in my personality is recognizable, and family members and friends frequently express their growing concern to Dan. I heavily despise this new normal and constantly search for answers, magic cures, for a rewind button. I want to go back to an earlier time in my life when I felt OK—not knowing that I was never actually OK and that I need to come completely undone before I can start putting the pieces back together again, a broken Humpty-Dumpty.

The delirium of insomnia sets in and my brain misfires rapidly, the neural pathways weak and unable to process information like they used to. Basic tasks become challenging; it takes over 30 minutes to pack school lunches because I am unable to focus on how to make a simple sandwich. The peanut butter and jelly containers stare mockingly at me as they sit on the counter whispering about my inadequacies as a mother. I walk the girls to school while a cardinal circles overhead, flaps its bright red wings, and chirps loudly at us, a gentle nudge reminding me that my spirit guides are indeed there and guiding me through this journey. After kissing the girls goodbye at the front doors of the school, I walk home and see at least 30 birds perched in a tree in the backyard, all of them staring directly at me. I cry out in desperation and beg them to help me.

I hop online and purchase a pricey Oura Ring, which collects and tracks data on biometrics that impact your well-being. It is supposed to provide insight into sleep cycles, blood oxygen, breathing regularity, body temperature, activity, and heart-rate variability. After two months of wearing this, it does not magically help me sleep and the only thing I gain is a smaller bank account and confirmation that I am not sleeping. I study the resulting output, certain that there must be an answer to my sleeplessness in the squiggly graphs. Staring at my computer screen makes me dizzy, and I lay my head down on crossed arms on my desk for a brief respite, reminiscent of the all-nighters I spent at the library during finals week of college, a quick recharge of the batteries to keep me going for another hour.

When I pick my head up, something that Psychic Stacy mentioned in our session last month flutters on the brink of awareness. I grab my journal and see "biomeridian testing" staring back at me in big block letters. I have no idea what this is, but it feels right. I research everything I can on biomeridian testing. It is a noninvasive alternative medicine technique used to assess the energy meridians of the body that can provide extensive information regarding underlying dysfunction and imbalances. It measures the body's electrical resistance at varying acupuncture points, bringing to light any food or environmental sensitivities, the functional status of organs, and what supplements may help bring your body back into alignment. I find someone who specializes in this practice a mere twenty minutes from my house and book an appointment.

Nine days later, I meet with a nurse practitioner, Nicole, at her holistic wellness clinic on the second floor of an old mall. A former plus-size model, Nicole has scarlet-red hair that beautifully contrasts with her bright-green eyes and porcelain skin. Her office has huge windows overlooking the parking lot, and cheerful sunshine pours in and bathes everything in a bright buttery glow, making it seem like summer in the dead of Wisconsin winter. She asks me to remove any jewelry before I lie down on the exam table and then proceeds to feel and massage all my extremities, palpate my knees, push on my stomach, and feel my spleen before directing me to sit down in a sizable weathered armchair next to her colossal oak desk.

We discuss the basic principles of biomeridian testing as I hold a copper pipe in my left hand while she sprays my right thumb with water before touching an electrode to the knuckle. I involuntarily recoil and pull my hand back, and she promises that I will not feel anything uncomfortable. The electrode is plugged in to her computer, which starts to emit sonar blips and sounds, like dolphins communicating underwater. The machine sends very small electrical currents through my body, and I do not feel a thing as the noises rise and fall with each mouse click and movement of the electrode. Nicole pecks furiously at her keyboard, takes copious notes, and makes annotations all over my chart. She checks each energy meridian in my body, and once we are finished an hour later, she discusses the results with me.

A look of concern crosses her face as she reviews and explains the resulting output. She is shocked by the multiple imbalances throughout my body and questions how I am still able to function on a daily basis. She starts with the good news: my liver is functioning well. The bad news: not only am I without a doubt dealing with a terrible case of chronic Lyme disease and parasites, but I also have Rocky Mountain spotted fever, Babesia, Bartonella, Ehrlichia, Mycoplasma, and mold toxicity. My hormone receptors are blocked, my lymphatic system is stagnant and sluggish, and my pituitary gland is troubled.

She explains that Lyme bacteria is quite stealthy, and while its usual form is in the shape of a spirochete, or corkscrew, when it is under attack, it curls up into a ball and protects itself with a biofilm, a slippery shield that protects it from the immune system and antibiotics, making it nearly impossible to kill. She stresses the importance of taking something to break down the biofilm before trying to eradicate the Lyme—otherwise, my efforts will be futile and useless. I mention the antiparasitic tinctures Dr. Nick recommended, and Nicole adds a few others to my arsenal.

I slump down into the overstuffed armchair in defeat, realizing that the mountain in front of me has just tripled in size. Seeing my reaction, Nicole leans over and gently squeezes my arm. She tells me she admires my resolve to find a way to heal, that Lyme presents a rare opportunity to find inner strength. She emphasizes the fact that natural treatments usually make you feel worse before you feel better and take a long time before you see real results, leaving patients frustrated and giving up too soon. She looks at me not with pity, but with respect, knowing that the battle I fight each day to reclaim my health despite the pain and uncertainty is not for the weak. It is the battle of a warrior.

CHAPTER 13

Basket Case

DECEMBER 2018

Parked in the church parking lot of Addy's school while mentally preparing to host the highly anticipated Christmas party for a classroom full of energetic three-year-olds, my phone buzzes with an incoming call, interrupting my breathing exercise. The phone has fallen out of my purse, and I scramble frantically to find it as it vibrates underneath bags of candy canes and pom-pom snowballs, glue bottles and jingle bells, causing them to rattle together in a discordant tune.

My stepmother is on the other end. "Sarah, it's Candy. Just wanted to check in and see how you're doing."

"I'm fine, just tired. Getting ready to host Addy's Christmas party in a few minutes so I can't talk long." I try to sound enthusiastic, my voice falling flat instead.

"I'm not sure how to say this, but your dad and I are worried about you. You haven't seemed like yourself lately and we get the sense that something is going on that you're not telling us. You've changed a lot these past few months, and you're withdrawing. We want you to know we are here if you want to talk. We love you very much." Her voice wavers slightly, tinged with discomfort at the verbal display of affection.

I laugh this off and keep things light, not wanting to get into a serious conversation minutes before the party.

"Yeah, thanks. I appreciate it, and you're right. I have changed. It's been a difficult few months with my health and I've been shifting, trying to figure out how to adjust to a new normal. But don't worry—I'm fine! Everything will be fine. I just need more sleep, that's all. I've got to run to the classroom now. Love you guys, too. Bye!"

As I end the call abruptly without waiting for her to respond, mascara rolls down my face from the tears that escaped, painting my cheeks black. I am upset with myself for not covering up my internal struggle as well as I thought, for not being stronger, for causing Dad and Candy to worry. As I gaze out my windshield at the cracked and faded asphalt, the overcast sky bloated with winter clouds waiting to unleash a fury of puffy lattice snowflakes, the grayness of the world matches the grayness inside me.

I surprise myself by contemplating leaving the parking lot and finding a road where I can drive my truck into an oncoming semi. I suddenly want to end it, all of it—the physical and the mental pain. I want an abrupt departure, to discard this wreck of a body, rid myself of the tortured anguish with a finality that closes out my story, rendering my last chapter complete. I don't want to hurt anyone else, just myself. Would I die right away from the impact, or miraculously survive only to become a vegetable, forcing Dan to make the unthinkable decision of when to pull the plug on my ventilator? Would my bones shatter, or would the airbags protect me, leaving nothing more than a smattering of colorful bruises? Death by semitruck leaves too many options open, too many unknowns. I need a more reliable alternative that leaves nothing up to chance.

The alarm on my phone startles me, alerting me that it is almost time to bring the joy and magic of Christmas to twenty eager children. I compose myself, ring the security bell to enter the school, and walk into the classroom with the happy face of a room mom who has created the perfect Pinterest party.

Room moms would normally bring in sugary snacks, whimsical cookies dripping in icing and dusted with red and green edible glitter, gingerbread men with chocolate chip buttons, and Capri Sun to wash it all down. They would help the kids insert the straws just right so as not to puncture through the foil pouches. My heavily restricted diet this year, however, causes me to fret about the food coloring and dye in processed nonorganic treats. I worry that the bioengineered ingredients will mutate the children's DNA and cause gene abnormalities later in life. I opt for organic Grinch fruit kebabs, topped off with a strawberry and mini marshmallow for the hat. My pulse races at the sugar content in the pristine white marshmallows, but they are organic, and it is Christmas, after all, so I throw caution to the wind. The drink of choice is a "melted snowman," petite water bottles decorated with two googly eyes and a red-ribbon scarf.

Addy welcomes me with an enthusiastic hug while my hands shake and tremble as I greet the other parent volunteers and instruct them how to run their activity stations. I'm certain they view me as an imposter, that they can see right through my fragile veneer while they silently judge the party I planned and the boring snacks to go along with it. The laughter and constant sounds of squealing joy pierce my ears and make my skin crawl like nails on a chalkboard. I stare at the wall clock and urge it to move faster as the secondhand ticks in slow motion, dragging the hour-long party into eternity.

I marvel at the stark contrast of life, the gap between the children's excitement and my thoughts of ending my life minutes prior.

The sky darkens with each minute of our drive home. The twinkling white icicle lights that dangle from the eaves and gutters of the houses reflect off the freshly fallen snow, making the ground sparkle and shimmer like a sea of diamonds. The nostalgic yuletide tunes on the radio are not nearly enough to elevate my holiday cheer or combat my dark thoughts. Addy chatters in her car seat happily, eagerly anticipating hanging her ornament on our tree with her sticky fingers that smell like peppermint from candy cane residue. I glance at her through the rearview mirror and smile meekly. My heart aches and bursts with love while knowing that I would welcome death with open arms and a smile.

While folding laundry several days later, the feeling of wanting to crawl out of my skin envelops me like the dark of night. It blankets me in despair. The indisputable realization that I will never be able to escape myself becomes too much to bear, and I hit myself in the face. My open palm strikes my left cheek and then the right, delicately at first and then increasing in intensity and frequency so quickly that I gasp, the sensation stinging both my face and hand. I am frantic, desperate for the brief respite the physical pain provides from the empty darkness inside, a hit of ecstasy that subsides just as quickly as it comes on, leaving me wanting more. I slap myself with passionate fury to shake this disease loose, get the Lyme spirochetes out of my brain, kill the parasites with the force of my hand. The pain feels like pleasure, the rush of adrenaline nauseatingly intoxicating, my palm and tender cheeks both flushed and angry.

The sensation of causing myself physical pain is familiar; it reminds me of the first time I cut the inside of my thigh with a blade, the grip of the white-and-aqua Gillette Sensor razor cushiony in my petite teenage hand. I cut myself to escape the pain of Mom's death, unaware that the satisfying sight of the bright-red droplets pricking my skin would never be enough to alleviate the emotional angst of the motherless daughter I had become.

The pain brings me back to my early twenties, drunk and alone in the shower, carving into my wrists with urgency, in a frenzied fervor after my brother's suicide. Unaware that there was a proper way to cut myself if I truly wanted to die, I would slice the skin off as if peeling a carrot, then watch the water mix with the blood gushing from the veins across my hand, drip down my fingertips, spiral into the drain like a tornado, whisking away my tears and platelets, cleansing and making me whole for a few seconds. One night cutting myself so deep in numb drunken violence, I was unsure my heart would be beating the next morning. I padded the open wound with gauze and Band-Aids and fell asleep with my arm above my head to staunch the bleeding. I woke up in agony the next morning with shame heavy on my heart, hiding what I'd done beneath bandages and long sleeves. I was strong enough to harm myself physically but too weak to ask for help.

A few months ago, gazing longingly over the balcony railing of a ninth-floor hotel room, I contemplated how long it would take for my body to splatter on the concrete pavers below. Three seconds? Two? I weighed the pros and cons of taking a running start to launch myself over versus climbing carefully to the outer edge and then letting go, swan-diving gracefully to the ground. Would my last moments be filled with euphoria or regret? What if I didn't die right away but wound up paralyzed, my mind still intact but my body even more broken, somehow escaping death and left to live out the rest of my miserable existence as an invalid? That would be poetic karma at its finest.

Aware that I am creeping into precarious territory again, I do not care. I bathe in the raw ache of my face, the dissipating tingle in my hand, the rush of painful pleasure. I want more. I walk into the kitchen, stare at the block of knives on the counter that whisper to me, that beckon me to pick them up. I feel the cool sharpness of their steely blades, daring me to see how much pressure is needed against my pale skin before drawing blood. Lost and spiraling, my trancelike state is broken by the playful shrieks of my daughters from upstairs. They snap me out of my reverie and remind me that I am a mother, and the crushing weight of being myself crashes down like a tidal wave.

CHAPTER 14

Into the Light

JANUARY 2019

A New Year should feel like a fresh start—the slate wiped clean with an entire 12 months rolled out like a sacred scroll, unsoiled and pristine, each 24 hours dedicated to creating a better version of myself. This year feels different. Somber, dull. The usual anticipatory excitement and thrill that accompanies removing the plastic wrap from the calendar, running my fingers over the glossy pages, and inhaling the inky smell fall short.

I stare at the numbered days in front of me that stretch out into infinity like a thin string of Silly Putty. I feel a mixed bag of emotions. The anniversary of Mom's death is January 2; she has been gone for 23 years, and the sadness is still there. I feel trapped by it. I mourn my mother and my teenage self who had to grow up too soon. Emotional coaching sessions with Islena have helped to unpack a great deal of this trauma but have only begun to scratch the surface of my wounds. She mentions a practice called The Emotion Code. I discover that a local practitioner is less than an hour away and immediately book an appointment.

The Emotion Code theorizes that 90 percent of physical ailments are due to trapped emotions or blocked energy, much of which has been carried with us from other generations, past events, traumas, abuse, or even experienced in the womb. If we are unable to feel the emotion and let it course through and out of our body, it becomes trapped and stays with us long after the event that caused it is over. Trapped emotions are tiny balls of energy stuck in the body that have a dramatic effect on thoughts, choices, reactions to situational stimuli, and they can impact bodily tissues and organs, causing physical and mental pain, self-sabotage, chronic fatigue, PTSD, and panic attacks. The trapped emotion is what disturbs overall balance and health.

Trained practitioners find and release these trapped negative emotions in the subconscious mind to protect us from further suffering. It is a simple yet transformative energy healing method. Science has come into agreement as well; epigenetics, quantum biology, and psychoneuroimmunology all have found that feeling positive emotions positively changes our biology at the cellular level and feeling negative emotions does the opposite, adversely impacting our body, mind, and spirit. I find this theory fascinating. Could my unconscious emotions be preventing true healing and actually be compounding my physical issues? Islena has certainly raised this connection during our sessions.

The drive to my initial appointment leaves plenty of time for me to question what I am doing, to second-guess myself and the validity of this practice. I also mull over what my father will think about this practice, how he will want to support my quest for healing but with disdain and doubt evident in his gaze and tone.

The door and sign for Wholesome Junction is nestled quietly within the multi-tenant office building, mysterious and clandestine, not wanting to draw attention to itself and only welcoming those who are meant to be there. Stepping inside the ground-level suite, I am greeted by the soothing sound of a tabletop waterfall fountain as the large droplets slowly snake down the faux stone façade and land quietly in a small pool of sandstone rocks. Taking a seat next to a green praying Buddha statue, I close my eyes and deeply inhale the faint scent of Frankincense permeating the air, listen to the calming melody of the peaceful spa music, and try to quell the tremors in my legs and arms.

A door creaks open down the dark hallway, then hushed voices and footsteps get louder as they approach. A tall, slender woman with tender blue eyes, perfectly aligned white teeth, and gray hair that holds lingering fragments of youthful brown at the ends, ushers out a prior client before turning toward me and introducing herself as Kathy. Her presence is delicate, ethereal; as we walk to her office she seems to hover just above the ground, floating rather than walking, her movement fluid and smooth.

She welcomes me into her dimly lit sacred office space and gestures for me to sit on the camel-colored suede sofa before sitting next to me, intimately close for someone I just met. Books line every shelf, chakra posters adorn the wall, and crystals and buddhas have been placed strategically throughout, leaving no surface untouched. Kathy asks what brings me to her today, and I reflexively burst into tears, the compassion radiating from her entire being making me feel safe, supported, and vulnerable.

"I've been sick, sad, searching for answers and meaning everywhere. Depression is overtaking me and I'm trying to fix myself by any means necessary."

Kathy smiles warmly and hands me a Kleenex. "I'm sorry to hear that, Sarah, and I look forward to diving into this further with you if you will let me."

Nodding my head in affirmation, Kathy gives me an overview of this practice, her training, and what a typical session consists of. She then asks to snip off a few locks of my hair and I nod again as I cringe, embarrassed as she touches the whispery thin strands. She places my hair on a glass plate, removes a pendulum from around her neck, holds it between her thumb and index finger, and dangles it over the glass. Her hand is steady, unmoving, and I watch in awe as the pendulum circles around the plate clockwise, then stops suddenly and changes directions, an innocent piñata at the mercy of the birthday child.

Kathy's hand is motionless as her torso slowly begins to rock back and forth and her eyeballs roll around behind her closed eyelids, each like a butterfly trying to escape its cocoon. Her voice changes as words stream out of her mouth in an odd baritone intonation, as though she has entered a different realm, as though someone else is talking through her.

The deep richness of this voice is strangely reassuring. "You are carrying emotions of many other generations as well as your mother's emotions that you picked up in the womb. Worthlessness, overwhelm, shock, confusion, humiliation, frustration, emotional and physical abandonment, grief, depression, panic, anxiety, fear. Did you have a traumatic birth or did your mother die in labor?"

I flatly reply, "I was adopted before I was born. My biological mother was young when she had me and never wanted children. She and my parents had a mutual friend, which is how they heard about me. Everyone was in the delivery room when I was born."

"Ahhh, that makes sense." She glances down at her notebook. "And what happened when you were fifteen or sixteen?"

"My adoptive mother died when I was sixteen. She had cancer, the long, slow, painful kind that took its time destroying her until finally killing her."

Kathy's face softens in empathy and interrupts my train of thought. "Sarah, you truly experienced the loss of two mothers—your biological mother when you were just a newborn, and then you lost your adoptive mother. Even though you were not consciously aware of what was happening, your soul knew what was going on in the womb. Your biological mother felt ashamed and embarrassed that she was pregnant at an early age, and your soul absorbed these feelings. There was also extreme guilt that she was not at a point in her life to raise a baby and was giving you up for adoption. The emotions you have been unintentionally carrying all these years have contributed to your illness. These have never been and are no longer yours to carry and we are going to work on releasing these today. These are your mother's emotions, and it is time to let them go."

I try to comprehend how an unborn baby can subconsciously hold emotions. I ask Kathy, "How exactly do you release these emotions for good?"

"Close your eyes and think of the earliest memory you have where you felt abandoned or unseen. You don't need to say it out loud but really try to go back to that moment in time."

She pauses for a minute while my mind travels backward, and I am shocked at what pops up, as it seems so insignificant.

I am four years old, sitting in our kitchen and waiting for lunch. My brothers, Mike and Matt, are sitting across from me on a yellow and orange Little Tikes plastic picnic table as my sister, Julie, naps in her baby swing. Mom and Grammy are arguing loudly over the proper way to cut hot dogs into mac 'n' cheese. Mom thinks they should be cut in circular slices, and Grammy thinks they should be cut in smaller pieces to avoid a choking hazard. Their arguing escalates as I tiptoe over and ask them to be quiet so as not to wake Julie. They both turn and yell at me to sit down, then continue their ridiculous argument.

"Do you have a clear visual of that memory?"

I nod and she continues. "I'm going to use this magnet and run it over your head and spine while you repeat after me."

I scoff. "A magnet?"

"Correct. Magnets are energy. Your body is energy. Just like a magnifying glass intensifies sunlight enough to start a fire, magnets act as an amplifier for the energy of your thoughts and emotions, enough to produce significant changes."

"All right, let's do it."

Kathy mumbles unintelligibly. I hear snippets of words—"fear," "anger," "grief"—and then meekly repeat after her when she instructs me to: "I am grateful for my mother. I am happy and healthy. I am loved and accepted. Love is why I am here. I am hopeful, optimistic, and joyful."

I say all of this three times while the magnet moves up and down, across my head and down my back, the metal inside removing the trapped emotions and wiping out my toxic subconscious programming, much like the hard drive of a computer being erased. There is a physical shift in my posture in addition to an emotional shift. I sit taller, shoulders squared, and I feel slightly stronger than moments before.

Once the magnet exercise is complete, she dangles her pendulum over the glass plate again and closes her eyes, listening to something only she can hear. Minutes pass before her eyes open and then she sets the pendant down and scribbles furiously in her notebook before looking up at me and inquiring, "What happened when you were twenty-four years old?"

I gasp out loud, then respond. "My brother killed himself playing Russian roulette." No matter how many times I have spoken these words over the years, it still feels surreal.

Kathy inhales sharply. "I see. This makes a lot of sense now as I am picking up feelings of terror and grief that began at age twenty-four. Your brother felt unsupported at that time in his life, and when he passed, his spirit energy of feeling unsupported was transferred to you. This happens quite often in sibling dynamics."

We repeat the magnet exercise as I echo Kathy's words back to her three times, words of affirmation, love, joy, and wholeness, in hopes that if I say them enough, I will start to believe them.

We quickly run over the allotted one-hour appointment, yet Kathy presses on. "You have severe excess adrenaline and cortisol, your endocrine system is imbalanced, and your skeleton is misaligned. There are severe issues with your lymphatic system, thyroid, adrenals, and kidneys. There is an alarming amount of heavy metal in your body, causing you to vibrate at a low level and feel a sense of despair and disconnection."

I stare at her in astonishment. "How do you know that? How can you possibly know that?"

Her blue eyes bore into mine. "My pendant never lies."

"That's incredible. I had a call with my doctor last week where he gave me updated protocol instructions for this month that focus on detoxing heavy metals from my body."

"I am merely providing you with what the pendant tells me. Everything is energy, and you have the power to change that energy, the power to create, the power to heal yourself. I also must mention that your spirit has left you. You have not been paying attention to it or listening to the warning signs, so it has abandoned you, causing you to project a will-to-die/no-will-to-live energetic broadcast, which has created a despair anchor in you."

I sob, finding it oddly comforting that she sees this and validates my pain all from a few strands of hair and a necklace.

She continues. "The negative energy state you have been vibrating in has attracted a lower astral entity that has been attached to you for some time."

Goosebumps erupt over my entire body. I am petrified to ask what this means yet do so anyway, bracing myself for what comes next. This sounds like something straight out of a horror movie.

"Lower astral entities are souls who have not yet crossed over to the other side, souls who are lost, scared, angry, sad. They're attracted to lower-vibrational people like moths to a flame."

"What? Am I possessed? Do I need an exorcism? This can't be real. How long has this thing been attached to me?" I claw at my arms and legs to remove this demon, this unwelcome, unseen, otherworldly presence that is using me without my knowledge or consent, another parasite.

Kathy firmly places her hand on my arm. "Calm down, it does not want to hurt you. I am going to remove this unwelcome entity, open your heart wall, and restore your spirit to your body."

I have no idea what she means, but I stay firmly rooted in place, too scared to move anymore. I feel Kathy slowly run the magnet up and down, up and down, up and down. She chants, using soft words to gently remove this lower astral entity from my body and send it back up to the light to be with God, to learn. It will only be welcomed back to this astral plane once it is ready to love. The low baritone of her voice vanishes, now replaced with a girlish timbre, a quiet murmur of something from above.

My insides quiver. There's a palpable stirring deep inside of me, the entity fighting back, resisting the pull of the higher power evicting it from my soul. Tears flow, emotions of every variety course through me, and for a fleeting moment, I feel like I am losing a dear friend. The sensation passes just as quickly, hitting me with a wave of relief and pure exhaustion.

Kathy opens her eyes, also clearly fatigued from the experience. She whispers in her own voice, "I think that is all for now. Make sure to drink plenty of water, journal, and rest. We did a lot of work today. Take some time to reflect and reach out if you have questions."

I wearily leave Kathy's office, shaky and unstable on my gray-Converse-clad feet, aware of every footfall in front of me. I sit in my truck before starting the engine. I'm incredulous, slowly absorbing and digesting, in disbelief yet also knowing what just happened was real as I cannot deny the lightness and renewed sense of hope coursing through me.

I drive home, desperate to stay in this peaceful glow forever. I am greeted at the back door by our faithful pit bull, Hailey, who exhibits more excitement than usual at seeing me. She does not leave my side for the rest of the day, sensing something different about me.

Mentally and physically depleted, I fall into bed that night and sleep soundly for the first time in months. The next day I wake up feeling refreshed, clear-headed, and, most importantly, alive.

CHAPTER 15

Losing My Religion

JANUARY 2019 – MARCH 2019

My coffee is piping hot, and I take tiny, cautious sips so as not to burn my tongue or scald the roof of my mouth. I close my eyes and inhale the salty warmth of the Caribbean air. I hear waves gently lapping along the coastline and enjoy the peacefulness of this moment. The serenity and lightness that has accompanied me since my session with Kathy falters a little, my tranquility punctuated by the deafening noise of a plane taking off from the small St. Maarten airport adjacent to our resort. Sleeping in is impossible here, and I relinquish all hope of catching up on sleep once again. The second-floor balcony of our hotel room provides an unrestricted view of the whalelike underbelly of the colossal 737 that climbs into the air, leaving plumes of jet fuel dancing across the atmosphere as its contrails cross with that of another jet to form a perfect white cross in the cloudless sky.

My gaze flickers between the sweeping view of the crystalline blue waters and the lush green courtyard below, where a woman is teaching sunrise yoga to a handful of guests, overachievers who like to work out while on vacation. Silent envy rises in my heart with wistful remembrance of the days when I felt good enough to exercise.

Walking to breakfast an hour later, Dan and I pass the yoga instructor, whose nametag boldly displays "Bianca" in large letters. We share the typical "Good morning, how are you? Have a great day!" pleasantries that strangers often say in passing, thinking nothing further of our brief exchange. The restaurant at our resort is suspended above a cliff overlooking Maho Bay, the impressive engineering of this complex architectural feat allowing for a once-in-a-lifetime dining experience. Basking in the glow of the warm Caribbean sun, we enjoy fruit and eggs while staring through the floorboards at the azure water crashing into the cliffs below before making our way to the spa lobby for a couples massage.

The frosted-glass doors open into a small yet welcoming waiting area, where we sip cucumber water and wait quietly in sunken white chairs, whispering softly to each other and flipping through magazines. Bianca appears, apparently serving as both the yoga instructor and spa manager, and greets us warmly. Up close, her energy is captivating, sparkling, joy radiating outward. The milky caramel complexion of her skin is accentuated by bright orange lipstick and pearly white teeth. Her positivity is infectious and draws me in.

She leads us back to the couples massage room, where the walls are painted a deep plum color and the soothing sounds of falling rain come from the hidden speakers. The inviting massage tables are draped in smooth white linens, and I instantly relax while lowering myself onto the heated bed and inhaling the scent of diffused eucalyptus oil. My nervous system is still haywire. Spasms and tremors reverberate throughout my body, my mind wanders, and I'm unable to focus. I tell myself to surrender, enjoy this next hour, relax. Letting out a deep exhale, I try to quiet my mind and simply notice my thoughts, acknowledge them, sit with them in full awareness. Psychic Stacy's words repeat in my head: "You need to have it out with God." Not fully knowing or understanding what this means, I ask the universe for help.

The hour goes by way too fast, and we emerge with our faces creased with wrinkles and our feet slippery in our sandals from the oil. Sunlight blinds our eyes as we step out of the dim serenity of the spa. Not quite back to our room yet, we hear urgent footsteps approach us from behind. I hear my name being shouted, and then I turn to see Bianca running toward me. She envelops me in a warm embrace once she reaches us, startling me with this random display of affection from a virtual stranger. Pulling out a small brown vial, she pours a few drops of its contents into her hands, rubs them together, and tells me to close my eyes and take three deep breaths in.

I do as instructed and inhale the sweet scent of oranges as she whispers in my ear, "Your solar plexus chakra is severely blocked. This will help open it. It is time to reclaim your power and have your voice be heard. You are stronger than you know."

My skin tingles. Is this a sign that the universe is actually listening to me? As I thank her profusely, tears prick my eyes at this kind soul whose message means more than she could ever possibly know.

We meet up with the rest of our work group who has already congregated at the pool. Portable speakers are pumping out '90s throwback tunes, and pina coladas and daiquiris are flowing with flamingo and unicorn inflatable drink holders bobbing next to their owners. I am surrounded by colleagues and strangers yet feel more alone than ever. The commotion and noise are too much for my nervous system. The multiple conversations blend into a disjointed symphony, making it impossible to focus, so I sneak away by myself to the nearby beach, telling Dan I need some alone time and I'll be back soon.

The sand is hot on my bare legs. The sun bakes them to a golden brown before turning them bright pink. Crystalline flakes of dried saltwater sparkle on my skin. Couples leisurely walk by, hands intertwined, eyes scanning the sugar-white sand for seashells and ocean treasures. I glower at their happiness through my tinted sunglasses, wondering what their lives are like and if they have ever experienced despair and pain like mine. The girlish laughter of tanned and toned college girls sunbathing nearby makes me feel even more alone. Their carefree attitude and conversation gets louder and more incoherent with each brightly colored umbrella drink.

Something gnaws at my soul, pushing up to the surface of my consciousness like scuba diver bubbles, and I feel the pulse of the earth beneath me. I am intimately connected with my surroundings; I sense every miniscule movement of the crabs scurrying out of their hiding holes as the water retreats and their frantic digging in the sand moments later to avoid the hungry seagulls circling overhead. I watch the flap of the gulls' alabaster wings in slow motion, hear the reverberation of their squawks, see every muscle in their webbed feet as they waddle, penguin-like, across the sand, each grain becoming distinct and separate from each other, a vista of individual iridescent particles.

Chronic illness is forcing me to reevaluate my belief system and reconsider the presence of God. After Mom died, I shunned my somewhat nontraditional Jewish upbringing. Having a Bat Mitzvah, attending temple and Hebrew school, and celebrating the high holidays coexisted with the Easter Bunny and a large Christmas tree to celebrate Dad's Catholic upbringing. Mom spearheaded our Jewish traditions and Dad complacently followed. I have fond memories of lighting the Menorah, spinning dreidels, and gagging at the smell of gefilte fish during Passover Seders. God died the day Mom did, and the last time I attended temple was at her funeral.

I am on the precipice of some monumental shift within but can't pinpoint it. It's like waking up from a vivid dream and losing all details the moment consciousness sets in. Not knowing what else to cling to in this moment other than a higher power, I feel like an AA attendee acknowledging the second step in the program. Succumbing to impulse, I lament and wail out, "Why won't you help me?" attracting concerned stares from strangers.

I slap the sand with my palms, kick at it with my feet, grunt and howl in agony and despair, a child throwing a temper tantrum. I have been living in the dark night of the soul for so long now and I am ready for the pain to stop. A gradual stillness washes over me as I stare at the relaxed waves rolling in and out, languid, unhurried, content and satisfied with their existence. Closing my eyes and turning my face directly to the sun like a young flower in bloom, I hear a voice respond, "I have never left you. You have all the answers you need. It is time to listen."

Two months later marks the 15th anniversary of Mike's suicide, and I reluctantly agree to attend a women's conference with my dear Lyme Warrior friend MK at a local church. She found God through her illness and healing journey, and her experience is paving the way for me. Her unwavering support and faith compel me to dip my baby toe back into the water of religion.

The expansive lobby is overwhelming. A sea of women is chatting and drinking free watered-down coffee, large smiles plastered on their faces in anticipatory excitement for the day. Standing there like a deer in headlights, unsure what to do or where to go, I spot MK and make my way through the crowd to her. She hugs me as we enter the large chapel and find our seats in a middle pew. The morning begins with an opening prayer and songs of praise, the melodies and energy in the room so beautiful that they move me to tears. Over 500 women sing together, "Death has lost its grip on me," and I feel a chain break, a sense of freedom and certainty that I will eventually find my way out of the darkness surrounding me.

One of the speakers discusses the four seasons, how each one serves a purpose and has a distinct reason, that God never abandons you and meets you in all seasons. She asks people to stand up when she calls out each season. As she says, "Winter," I stand up slowly, ashamed and embarrassed, my face beet red, certain the entire room is staring at and judging me. MK grabs my hand and gives it a light squeeze.

The speaker continues. "Winter is hard, cold, dreary. You may not see the light for days, but it doesn't last forever. Spring always follows, a renewal and resurrection. Plants that have been dormant and underground in the dark bloom once again, stronger and prettier than ever."

Glancing timidly around the chapel, I see numerous women standing, and realization dawns on me that there is commonality and community in being vulnerable and openly showing others our pain, our shadow, our sorrow, even if it's just by standing together in silence. Frequently caught up in my own pain, it's difficult to comprehend that others are suffering too. Looking around the room provides a new sense of understanding that so many others are facing demons and dealing with their own battles.

We adjourn for lunch before the breakout sessions. The irony of today's date is not lost on me. The heaviness and constant thoughts of my brother echo in the back of my mind, and I attend a session on dealing with traumatic loss.

Pastor Mel, a soft-spoken grandfatherly figure with a shock of white hair and deep sadness in his bright cobalt eyes, walks to the podium and clears his throat loudly, nervousness evident in his gently trembling hands. His adult daughter passed tragically years prior and the powerful words he shares today resonate deeply among the packed room.

"Death is a severe and abrupt ending," he says, "an absolute dividing line with zero room for negotiation or repair. You are stunned into numbness, gazing straight ahead at the pain with nothing but quiet hours of reflection alone with your thoughts. Survival is primal and physical in those early days of loss as you grapple with a harsh new reality."

Women cry silently, nod their heads in agreement. All of us are bonded together by our shared losses.

"The definition of survival is to live or exist despite difficult circumstances. The deep pain of loss always comes from something good, from a deep love. Would you rather have had your loved one for the amount of time you did or not at all?"

I have never thought about my circumstances from this perspective. Would I rather have had Mom for 16 years or not at all? Would I rather have had Mike for 22 years or not at all? Some modicum of health for 37 years or not at all? I have been angry for so long, focusing on the unjustness of it all, on the shitty hand I was dealt, on the loss and the abandonment and the sickness, when I should have been focusing on the in-between, the happy moments, the laughter, the rest of my family, my loving children and husband.

Pastor Mel continues. "Think of your life as a plant. Plants need to be pruned, and branches trimmed back to create more growth and beauty. There is a purpose to pruning so the plant will be even more fruitful. We don't always understand why God trims certain branches, but we need to trust that he is doing so to create something even more magnificent."

Reflecting upon the messages of today, it dawns on me that if God truly does exist, perhaps he does not mean to rescue or help us; perhaps he uses our trials and tribulations to transform us. I now understand what Psychic Stacy meant by doing the spiritual work. Perhaps chronic illness is shaping my soul and forming the foundation of my spiritual growth.

CHAPTER 16

Save Me from Myself

MARCH 2019

My hair continues to fall out by the handful. I dread taking a shower and use only one pump of shampoo and conditioner instead of the usual three. The once full and vibrant strands are now flimsy and thin. They delicately tickle my legs as they slide down and into the floor drain. I consider shaving my head, ripping off the Band-Aid instead of tugging it slowly and drawing out the agony. Too embarrassed to go to my usual salon, I ask Dan to cut my hair, which he reluctantly agrees to. We stand in silence and listen to the snipping of the scissors as my split ends flutter soundlessly to the floor.

Of all the symptoms, hair loss is quite minimal compared to others, but it's one of the most difficult to cope with mentally. Losing my hair feels like losing part of my identity. Always long and thick, it has been an armor to protect and beautify me, a shield to put in front of my face and conceal my insecurities. Now I am fully exposed and on display. There is little to hide behind or flick nonchalantly to the side when I am nervous. Although my emotions are healing and my spiritual faith is growing, my physical body is still suffering.

Vanity gets the best of me, and I scour the internet for local hair-loss clinics, attend informational meetings on surgical options, and listen to sleazy, unqualified multilevel marketing greaseballs pitch me on hair replacement gels, creams, lotions, and pills that promise to provide thicker, fuller hair in only a month. I make an appointment for an initial consultation with Marcia, a wig lady, whose website touts her compassion and understanding of every client's unique situation.

I park on the ground level of an old shopping center and scan the parking lot to see if anyone is watching me, like I'm a celebrity avoiding paparazzi, as if complete strangers care about the intimate details of my life. Taking the decrepit concrete steps two at a time down the staircase to the lower level, I stop in front of a hazy glass door, clouded over from neglect and time. As I push it open and walk into the stale room, a familiar smell hits me and takes me back in time to my Aunt Clara's basement when she and Grammy would color each other's hair once the gray began to peek through. The chemical smell of hair dye mixed with old-lady perfume permeates the air and infiltrates my nostrils like smoke.

Marcia is camouflaged among the rows of eerie mannequin heads and startles me when, eyeing me warily, she curtly asks, "May I help you?"

"Yes, we spoke on the phone. I'm Sarah, here for our appointment?"

The caginess in her eyes is unnerving, making me feel like I'm doing something wrong, like I'm somewhere I shouldn't be. She leads me to a salon chair, and my butt is barely in the seat before she slams her foot on the hydraulic pump to raise me up.

"Why are you here, Sarah?" Her tone is punitive and accusatory, as though she is doing me a favor and I am unworthy of her time, a mere peasant in the presence of the royal queen.

My face turns red hot before I sheepishly respond, "Well, my hair has been falling out for the past year and a half. I'm scared that one day I will wake up bald, and I want to be proactive to see what options are out there."

She scoffs. "You still have a full head of hair. The people I see are cancer and alopecia patients who've lost much more hair than you have. Sure, your hair is fine and could be thicker, but I wouldn't worry about it. Are you getting enough sleep? Are you stressed? Do you have a healthy diet? All of these can affect your hair growth."

I instantly hate this woman, resent her callousness and insensitivity. "I'm aware that I still have hair, and yes, I fully understand all the things that impact hair growth. Working with doctors and specialists has not mitigated the hair loss. It feels like I have one strand of hair left and I just want help."

The last few words get stuck in my throat as I don't want to express to this cold-hearted woman how terrified I am that if I lose all my hair, I will ultimately lose myself, become less of a woman. I question if Dan will still love me with no hair and if my kids will look at me differently. When Mom lost her hair, of course we still loved her, but there was also an element of embarrassment to being the only teenager whose mother had cancer and was bald. I immediately feel guilt for all these thoughts, that something as vain as my hair or lack thereof would change Dan's or my children's love for me, that it could have any impact on my self-worth.

Marcia softens ever so slightly, seeing my discomfort. She grabs several hairpieces and wigs for me to try on, but I am already checked out. I hop down from the chair, discouraged and once again questioning my sanity. I thank her brusquely for her time and storm out of there, the sickening scent of her suite glued to my clothes for the rest of the day.

The moon peers at me through the narrow slits of the blinds like a peeping Tom, taunting me with its increasing roundness, forewarning me that it will be full in 72 hours. I dread its majestic beauty; my increase in symptoms coincides perfectly with each day's expansion of the pregnant white orb. Dr. Nick recommends that I double my dosage of antiparasitics and push my body and mind to the limit to really attack them this month. I am holding on for dear life as I thrash my legs and arms wildly to quiet their movement and allow me to get some broken sleep.

Morning comes way too early. Opening my eyes, I am overcome with disorientation, vertigo. I can't decipher where I am—a hotel room, someone else's house? Am I still dreaming or am I awake? What day is it? What time is it? Only after several minutes does the fog recede and I recognize my bedroom, the dark espresso of the dresser and cloudy-gray comforter no longer strangers but friendly faces. I gingerly get out of bed, throw on some sweats, and wake the children. I get them dressed, fed, and Nolan and Everly off to school. I walk home with Addy to put a movie on before her nap, praying she will sleep instead of crawling out of her crib.

Today needs to be focused on detoxing as much as possible. I pour boiled distilled water into a French press, the toffee-colored coffee grounds swirling through the glass like a tornado, letting it steep and cool before straining four cups of liquid into a large glass measuring cup and adding a teaspoon of blackstrap molasses for the perfect enema recipe. Setting the solution on the bathroom counter for later, I turn the infrared sauna on and gather towels, coconut oil, the enema bucket and hoses, and dry brushes for the full detox experience.

Addy and I sing songs and rock gently in the squeaky rocking chair before her nap. I sprinkle Mommy dust on her and close the door, then shift my eyes to the baby monitor and watch her play with the tag of her lovey and tail of her stuffed giraffe before she drifts off into peaceful slumber.

Stripping all my clothes off, I run the coarse bristles of the dry brush down my arms, up my legs, and in a circular motion across my stomach where my C-section scar and slight paunch are now permanent fixtures since having kids. Dry brushing exfoliates the skin, increases blood flow, and promotes lymphatic drainage, helping to eliminate waste and toxins from the body. After five minutes of this, I zip myself into the portable infrared sauna and stare outside at the dirty snow and the barren maple tree in the backyard, keenly aware that no birds have perched there recently and hoping they survived the recent bitter temperatures.

Replaying the experience at the wig store in my mind upsets me, makes me wonder if the hair loss is another physical manifestation of emotional wounding and a malfunctioning nervous system. I have done so much over the past nine months, and it does not seem to be enough, the end nowhere in sight; am I seeking an external solution to an internal problem?

Eckhart Tolle's words echo in my thoughts: "I cannot live with myself any longer. Am I one or two? If I cannot live with myself, there must be two of me: the 'I' and the 'self' that 'I' cannot live with. Maybe only one of them is real." I ponder this, trying to wrap my head around this existential musing, and get lost in a circular thought pattern like the chicken and egg paradox.

Dripping with sweat that reeks of pure ammonia and stings my eyes, I am sufficiently overheated and flushed as I enter the second half of my detox ritual. The coffee solution is cool enough now, still pleasantly warm yet not scalding. Before lying on the ground and lubing the hose up with coconut oil, I scroll through my phone, looking for something that will distract me and get me out of this mental funk.

Dr. Nick recently sent me a link to a podcast he did with one of his colleagues, Dr. Scott, on the power of the mind, which seems fitting for this very moment. Closing my eyes and opening my asshole, I let their words and the coffee in.

"Many chronically ill patients unintentionally categorize themselves as victims and get stuck in a vicious feedback loop of negativity, both contributing factors why full healing and recovery cannot be achieved." Being sick for so long, I blame myself. I reflect on all my mistakes and missteps, certain I brought this on, I created this illness. My victim mentality has created incessant worrying and a self-labeling nomenclature of *my* symptoms, *my* chronic Lyme disease, *my* hair loss, *my* parasites, *my* lack of health.

I focus on the words from the podcast:

After three months, chronic infection and illness are processed and perceived by a different part of your brain. Mindset is everything—your cells are listening all the time. The brain is like a muscle; muscles need to be constantly worked, challenged, torn, and repaired to get stronger. There is more going right in your body than there is going wrong, no matter how bad you feel. Pain is inevitable but suffering is not; suffering occurs when you believe a thought that argues with what is, with the truth. There is always a choice; you define your own suffering.

Healing does not happen all at once; it happens by making a dent, by chipping away slowly but surely. It never happens as fast as we would like but that does not mean it is not occurring. There is no quick fix, no magic pill. Deep and permanent healing requires relinquishing control, surrendering fully, letting the body and mind do what they innately know how to do. If treating the physical body alone does not resolve symptoms, then maybe the body alone is not what caused it.

Lyme disease has become my entire being, defining my existence, but listening to the messages throughout this podcast makes me realize it does not have to, that it does not constitute who I am or my worth as a person. Telling myself that I don't feel good because of *my* Lyme is preventing true healing. Not having *my* health and being in constant pain has diminished everything, has made me see through the tunnel-vision lens of illness like a horse with blinders, blocking out all the beauty. It is time to remove those blinders and create purpose from my pain, to use what is happening to me to help someone else.

Logically, this makes sense. Reality is a different story; however, I make up my mind in this moment to reframe my perspective, to think not about why this is happening to me, but why this is happening *for* me. This is an opportunity to forever change my knowledge and perception of who I am, a crucial crossroads where I will either lose myself and waste away into nothingness or I will find myself and come out changed, more resilient than ever. Nobody can save me from myself except myself.

CHAPTER 17

Wonderwall

DECEMBER 1995

"Who are you?"

I must read her cracked lips, as nothing more than a wet wheeze escapes her mouth.

The usual softness of her familiar brown eyes has disappeared; they are no longer hers. They've been replaced with those of a feral animal backed into a corner, wild with terror. The hole in her neck is the size of a quarter, a giant tracheostomy tube protruding from it so she can breathe, dried yellow mucus crusted around the edges. Two EMTs restrain her, delicately weaving their way among the tubes and wires, around the colostomy bag of urine and waste that hangs from her side. They tie her flailing arms and legs to the railings of the stretcher, and I hold on to the door handle for stability as we barrel down the highway. Dad zigzags in and out of traffic behind us to keep up.

Time slows down as the ambulance speeds up. The flashing red lights and high-pitched wail of the siren are unable to silence the deafening noise of those words.

"I'm your daughter, Mom."

The last six years catch up to me in this instant and I detach from myself, die inside at this precise moment. I am unable to comprehend that my own mother cannot recognize me, that she views me as a stranger. My mind floats away to avoid the unforgiving reality of this night, the pain slicing back and forth through my heart like a crosscut saw.

The months leading up to this night are brutal—for Mom and our entire family. Chemotherapy, radiation, and cancer drugs annihilate her cognitive function, extinguish her years of radiology and medical school training in a matter of months, turn her brain into a delusional hallucinogenic wasteland. Moments of lucidity seldom arise, but when they do, she attempts to communicate with us using a marker and a whiteboard. Her once neatly spaced loopy cursive is now a string of scribbles like a one-year-old coloring for the first time.

My three siblings and I take turns sitting with her, keeping watch when the day nurses leave and before Dad gets home. We help her to the portable commode adjacent to the eyesore of a hospital bed in the middle of the bedroom. We are too ashamed to help her wipe, and we avert our eyes in embarrassment to allow a small modicum of privacy. Her coughing fits terrify me; she gasps for air through the hole in her neck as though she is drowning. She spews greenish-brown phlegm onto her gown and blanket. I wipe away as much as I can and sigh deeply when it is over, my heart returning to a normal rate once she falls back into a restless sleep.

Relief floods through me every time Dad gets home, my fear of being alone in the room with her slowly subsiding with each footfall of his on the steps. I am in the hallway before he can reach the bedroom door, impatient to escape the smell of sadness and death.

Not knowing what to say or do, my dad, siblings, and I avoid talking with each other about our feelings. We tiptoe around the fact that our cancer-riddled matriarch is peering over the precipice of death, becoming friends with the Grim Reaper who has taken up permanent residence at her bedside.

Mom stood up this tragic night, a final burst of adrenaline coursing through her body. Her stubbornness and determination took over for a few minutes as she swatted at the tubes and cords like they were gnats, pulled and tugged at the trach in her throat that supplied oxygen to her lungs. Her gown came untied, fell from her shoulders, and left her fully exposed, her skin hanging from her gaunt stomach like an oversized apron. She stumbled and fell to the floor in a naked heap. My father and brother rushed into the room upon hearing the commotion. They lifted her gently then placed her back on the bed, held her down, and pulled her weak arms through the holes of her stained gown. The minutes passed like hours, expanded and dilated like pupils. The ambulance arrived and we all watched as she was carried downstairs on a stretcher, babbling incoherently and shooting daggers through her eyes at the EMTs. Dad yelled at me in a panic to get in with her and told me that he would follow the ambulance in his car and meet us in the emergency room.

Dad and I sit with her for hours that night. We are unmoving, silent, glued to the cold plastic of the hard chairs. We stare at the colorful twinkle lights and silvery snowflake ornaments that adorn the tiny tree on the nurses' station and listen to the Christmas music that plays softly over the fuzzy hallway speakers.

Mom dies in a sterile hospital room in hospice care two weeks later.

My siblings and I retire to our own bedrooms upon hearing the news to grieve in private, like a proper family does. I sit at my ink-stained white desk, tears dotting the pages of my journal, and do the only thing that feels right—I write.

That cold, starry night, the ambulance whisked you away.
I was by your side, the memory still painful to this day.
You were so scared; you didn't recognize me.
That was only the drugs, I now clearly see.
As your husband—my father, and I sat crying,
I couldn't help to think that you would soon be dying.
This thought caused much pain and sorrow.
I thought how free you would be, come tomorrow.
This disease took you from us, with no definitive start.
And you took along a piece of my heart.

How does life go on without your mother? At a time when you both need and despise her the most, when you are no longer a girl, but not quite a woman? Guilt and blame engulf me for her premature departure. Perhaps if I had been a better daughter, listened more, helped more, loved her more, she would still be here.

Our house slowly fills with muted sounds of sympathetic condolences and the aroma of overcooked brisket and noodle kugel casseroles. I crack open my door and listen to hushed voices: "She's in a better place." "Please let us know what we can do." "I loved her like a sister." "We're all here for you."

My eyes dry up, and I put on a comfortably numb nonchalant façade like armor, walk down the stairs to accept hugs and looks of pity, and tell everyone I am fine, that I have homework to complete before English class tomorrow, as though this takes precedence over my mother's death.

Mom's dear friend Idy tsks. "Oh, Sarah, you don't need to worry about that. The teacher will understand. You take as much time off from school as you need."

Adamant that I must complete an essay on how Fitzgerald uses symbolism and irony in his great American novel, I write in my spiral notebook on our faded leather couch, tune out and ignore the sadness around me, edit and polish my essay, and turn it in to Mr. Glaznap the very next day.

Adjusting to life without Mom is awkward, like puberty. Best friends become strangers, and I misinterpret their abrupt distance and lack of knowing what to say as not caring. Students boldly stare for far too long as I walk through the hallways, pointing and whispering. My status quickly turns to that of an outcast, a leper, as if associating with me will cause cancer to spread to their mothers as well.

No longer having a table full of friends to eat with in the cafeteria, I hide in the library between rows of Encyclopedia Britannica volumes. As the librarian walks by, I shove my wilted sandwich into my backpack and bury my nose in a textbook, pretending that precalculus is fascinating—why in the world aren't there more students in here reading about derivatives and limits of a quotient? The usual carload of friends that fill my truck after school has dwindled. I chain-smoke Marlboro Reds alone while listening to 2Pac and Biggie, and enter our empty forlorn shell of a house, a skeleton of a formerly happy home.

The kitchen is lifeless, devoid of snacks and my mother's warm welcome, and I retreat to the comfort and safety of my bedroom as the late-afternoon daylight falters and the winter sky darkens. Tacky, colorful, ginormous bulb Christmas lights hang like lanterns across my window, dousing the room in an unnatural glow and muting the pain of loss with forced ambiance.

The hallway phone sits quietly on my bed, its cord loose and droopy from being carelessly stretched. No one calls to check on me or invite me to hang out. The phone mocks me with its silence, makes me check to ensure the ringer is still on (of course it is). I sink deeper into my difference and outcasted-ness, a deep knowing settling into my bones that I am not like the rest of the students in high school. I am tarnished and alone, a motherless daughter carrying the burden of shame and embarrassment that hangs around my neck like an albatross.

The rock band Oasis blasts through the speakers of my six-disc CD player for hours on repeat. "Wonderwall" drowns out my tears, making me wish that someone would be the one that saves me.

I push the pain down as far as it will go. I use anything to avoid feeling it—boys, cigarettes, weed, alcohol, razorblades—and ignore it. I pretend I got over her death in a matter of weeks. I "stay strong" for the sake of my family. Gravitating toward boyfriends who are not good for me, I act out in ways my mother would be ashamed of. I use them the same way they use me. I feel the wrongness of it while clinging desperately to them to fill the void in my broken heart. My reliance on them is unhealthy but necessary. Their attention and love give me validation, purpose, and a reason to live, helping ensure my survival. They become my entire world, an all-consuming distraction, yet I cannot let them in fully for fear they may leave me and cause more pain. I am physically there but emotionally unavailable. The breakups are so devastating that it feels like another death until I move onto the next relationship days later.

Twenty-one years later, Lyme disease is forcing me to finally deal with and grieve Mom's death properly. Unburdening the years of stored pain onto the listening ears of my emotional coach, Islena, is difficult yet cathartic. Our work together helps me realize that bypassing the grieving process and burying emotions has contributed in part to my weakened immune system and made me more susceptible to getting sick. She's taught me that the root of many chronically ill patients is due to emotional blocks.

Islena quickly uncovers emotional patterns that I forged through my fires of loss, patterns that existed prior to any of my physical ailments. Staying busy has long been my neurological response when uncomfortable feelings arise, short-circuiting my normal human function of emotional processing when under duress. The human brain is designed to repeat familiarity. My habitual reaction of avoiding difficult feelings that was imbued in me at such a young age is now my default response, even in situations when it is inappropriate.

Cutting people out of my life entirely is easier than having a difficult conversation when conflict arises. Running away and isolating from meaningful friendships protects me from any potential future hurt. Drinking too much numbs the sadness momentarily but causes it to violently erupt when the alcohol takes over. Cycling on and off Prozac makes life tolerable and dulls both the good and the bad. My personality has been shaped by trauma and death, which have molded my communication style into an aggressive abruptness with a hint of direct dismissiveness.

Islena points out that my knee-jerk reactions are no longer appropriate. The self-abandonment and devaluation of my own worth have run their course, and it is time to make meaningful changes if I want to heal. I hate that she is right, that she can read me like a book and always has the answers.

We spend months working together to retrain my brain, form new neural pathways, and create a new response mechanism with more productive outcomes at this stage in my life. Changing my brain wiring and neuroplasticity is like going to the gym. Muscle mass only increases when I lift weights repeatedly. Gains are not visible after only one gym session—they're built slowly, through consistency and repetition. Thought patterns only begin to change when I notice them, acknowledge them, and choose to react a different way, time and time again.

Awareness is the first step. Acknowledging the old familiar patterns when they arise is difficult at first but becomes more comfortable with practice. I talk to myself and say out loud that these patterns are no longer relevant and no longer serve me. I change the programming in my head to *I am valuable. I am worthy. It is safe to feel hard emotions and let them pass through me.* Releasing the pain, feeling the feels, and blessing the past will result in true emotional clarity and freedom.

I didn't relate to Mom as much before I became a mother myself and fell ill. Now I empathize with what she went through; I can see through the lens of a dying 49-year-old mother instead of the lens of a lost 16-year-old daughter. I better understand the sacrifices she made, how hard she worked to provide for us, how much she loved us. I admire her for the strength it took to still show up for us amid her cancer. I am sorrowful for the guilt she inevitably had for leaving her husband with four children, and I take solace in knowing a woman at the end of her life makes peace with a lot of things.

Islena takes me back in time like a hypnotist to talk to my inner child—the young part of my psyche that influences my adult thoughts and reactions, the emotionally stunted 16-year-old Young Sarah. Islena has me drop awkwardly into my younger self and place my hand over my heart to truly feel the depths of despair and grief in those initial months following Mom's death. My stone façade topples like Jenga blocks with her soothing words and empathy, the once solidly stacked blocks now teetering on the brink of collapse, the pain flowing out of me through my salty tears.

Anger occasionally arises within me toward Islena. I am irritated with her for challenging everything I have ever known, for taking me outside my comfort zone, for asking the hard questions, making me explore the darkest shadowy corners of my mind. At times I resist and refuse to speak as Islena and I stare at each other, Young Sarah dominating Adult Sarah and taking over in stubborn defiance. Understanding that my younger self is showing up and exasperated that my adult self cannot properly reparent her on my own, I am frustrated that I must still deal with something that happened more than twenty years ago.

Adult Sarah pushes through, however, and joins Young Sarah. She holds her hand, taking care not to admonish or discount her grief and holds space for her instead. She thanks her for stepping up and helping her flailing family. Assures her that she had no control over Mom's health, that the subconscious blame and historical shame she has been carrying all these years has never been and is no longer hers to carry; she has been blaming herself for something she is blameless for.

The visceral response I have to this inner-child work and pushing on this years-long wound makes me want to run, and for the first time, I do the opposite. I stand in my discomfort, let it wash over me, through me, and feel the smallest stirring of a welcome sense of lightness and closure.

CHAPTER 18

One Call Away

MARCH 2019

In typical Wisconsin fashion, Mother Nature blesses us with a fierce snowstorm that blankets the ground with nine inches of snow in less than twelve hours, then graces us with arctic temperatures and wind chills that plummet into the double-digit negatives, forcing schools to close. The harshness of the bitter cold is offset by the glittery glow of the hoarfrost that sparkles from the trees and ground, turning the landscape into a delicate and ethereal shimmering fairy land.

In the morning, the internal clock of the children rouses them, and they stumble drowsily into my room, their sleep-crusted eyes widening with excitement when I tell them school is cancelled. We lie in my bed, enveloped in the warmth of the comforter and our morning breath, and I want to stay glued to this peaceful coziness all day. Staring outside at the blinding snow, I notice the interior corners of the windows have gathered ice flowers overnight. Exquisite, freshly sculpted works of art are etched on every window like Elsa's private garden, fractal patterns resembling ice feathers and ferns. I haven't enjoyed a moment like this in quite some time, but the magic is soon interrupted by urgent requests for breakfast and hot cocoa.

Dan is in Chicago for a conference. His presence and help with our children are sorely missed as my tolerance and patience are still thin. My fuse is short and easy to light while I adjust to this month's updated protocol and supplement schedule following my monthly call with Dr.

Nick. The alarm on my phone chimes every few hours, a shrill reminder to take a portion of my 54 daily supplements and droppers full of 11 herbal tinctures. I'm always on edge and off-kilter when adding in new formulas to my protocol, so I know today is going to be painfully long, that each symptom will be exacerbated and intensified as the new supplements go to war with the bacteria running amok inside me. I can do hard things, and I steel myself to deal with the onslaught of symptoms accompanied by the screaming of excited children.

Settling the girls onto the couch to watch a movie after breakfast, I slowly clean up the spilled milk, stray Cheerios, and sticky residue from syrupy waffles like a robot, a machine functioning on autopilot, detached and going through the motions to ensure survival. I reflect on the redundancy of my days: pills, dishes, fatigue, cleaning, Barbies, enemas, emails, laundry, snacks, sauna, dog shit, Legos, pills, pills, pills.

While a cartoon crab sings animatedly about life under the sea, my brain sinks to the depths of self-loathing like waves flowing back to the ocean at low tide, proudly displaying the debris and ugliness that only hours before was hidden by the water. I pray for high tide to come and drown out my inadequacies, make me feel whole for a few moments. Afraid of being alone with the kids for the long hours that stretch out in front of me and wanting to shelter them from my erratic and unpredictable mood swings, I call my father.

The thought of preparing a home-cooked meal puts me into a frenzied panic, so I brave the slippery streets and subzero temperatures with the girls to meet Dad out for dinner—the road conditions much less frightening than cooking. The mountains of snow have been plowed to the side of the streets and trucks are scattering large salt rocks behind them like Hansel and Gretel leaving a trail of breadcrumbs. Although more tables are empty than usual, the restaurant is bustling, and we are seated in a quiet booth off to the side. Normally I'd order a glass of white wine, but the unease I feel tonight makes me opt for a club soda with a lime. After placing our order, the girls happily get lost in their iPads with their headphones on, presenting a rare opportunity for Dad and me to talk one-on-one.

We have always had a good father-daughter relationship (apart from a few teenage years), but our dynamic changed once I got sick and began exploring alternative healing methodologies. A Stanford and University of Wisconsin Medical School graduate, Dad is a highly sought-after orthopedic surgeon who specializes in sports medicine and commands a great deal of respect in and out of the operating room. His education in Western medicine leaves little room for acceptance or understanding of holistic healing, and prior conversations about both my physical and mental health created friction between us, an unspoken awkwardness that we have danced around to avoid upsetting one another.

There is a different feel to the energy tonight, however—a weightiness hovering between us like a heavy perfume. Call it paternal instinct, gut feeling, or intuition, Dad senses that something is off with me.

"What's going on with you, Sarah? You haven't been yourself for a while and I'm concerned."

I take a deep breath, intent on keeping it together so the girls won't see me cry. "I'm concerned too. Lyme has turned my world upside down, shattered it into a million little pieces, and I feel broken. I'm trying to find a way to put myself back together but I'm not quite sure how. I question my meaning and purpose, the reason for existing. I'm scared I'm going to wind up like Mom."

Dad leans in, a deep resolve in his eyes. "Sarah, you are not broken. You are in the process of discovering who you are and who you are meant to be. You have always been unrelentingly hard on yourself, and I encourage you to be more forgiving, more compassionate. Talk to yourself like a good friend would. Accept your faults and mistakes and learn from them."

"Yeah, I guess," I say. "I know you're not a believer in Eastern medicine, but I sense deep down that this path will help me heal fully, that part of the reason I am so sick is due to the thoughts running rampant through my head."

"Just because I don't believe in something doesn't mean it can't work. Facts, science, operating, and fixing patients' fractured bones is all I've ever known. I am in your corner no matter what. I will never judge you for trying unconventional methods. All I want is for my daughter to be healthy again."

His words of encouragement buoy me, a life raft of support, and prompt me to regale him with stories of all the crazy things I have been doing—coffee enemas, infrared sauna, light therapy, salt rooms, colonics, reiki, sound baths, tapping, celery juice, eating whole garlic cloves as if staving off a vampire attack.

Dad chuckles his deep belly laugh as I continue. "I also know you're suspicious of psychics, but I have seen several and recently saw a genuine energy healer. Getting sick has brought out the worst emotions in me, and she's helping me uncover subconscious blocks and release them."

"What do you mean by that?"

"I thought I fully processed the deaths of Mom and Mike years ago, but there is still unresolved trauma and emotional damage stored in my body from this that I need to work through."

Saying these words out loud to my father makes me realize for the first time in my life that I never once put myself in Dad's place or considered how his life was impacted. Immature and young, cloaked in my own grief like a burial shroud, I was oblivious that my father and siblings were suffering too.

Dad's shoulders sag, thoughts of Mom and Mike still haunting him too. He says, "I was so angry with your mother for dying and leaving me with four children to raise on my own. Only now, years later, can I acknowledge that this was grief manifesting as anger. My hair loss started shortly after Mom died due to stress and then worsened with Mike's passing, so I understand the physical toll that emotions have. Our family has experienced more than our fair share of death and loss. None of you kids are allowed to die before me—I already experienced the loss of one child and I couldn't bear the loss of another."

I gasp, the suicidal thoughts from a few weeks prior still lingering in the back of my mind like the smell of burnt popcorn. Awareness dawns on me that if I ended my life, my pain would only be transferred onto others, onto my father, and I cannot bear the thought of that.

"I'm so sorry, Dad. I never stopped to think about your feelings over all these years of pain. As a child, I thought you and Mom were superheroes. Once she died, I couldn't think about anyone else's perspective or look at life through your lens. For what it's worth, you did a great job raising us, and now that I'm a parent, I understand and appreciate the sacrifices you made and how hard you worked to provide for us."

His eyes well up. "I still question if I did enough with my life. Did I help enough patients? Was I a good-enough surgeon? A good-enough father? A good-enough husband? Could I have done more? I remember how hard it was to lose my parents, and I was in my fifties with four children and a flourishing career. I had to make the ultimate decision on when to pull the plug on my dad, a choice I hope you never have to make. My parents were always a safety net for me, one call away. Although they lived halfway across the country in California, just knowing they were there was comforting. Losing Mom for all of you kids at such a young age was very traumatic. She and I parted on good terms, and we had time to say everything that needed to be said."

We are interrupted by the arrival of our entrees and the magic between us evaporates, but the door of communication is left ajar. There is a palpable shift in our relationship, this conversation more authentic than any, making me feel supported and heard.

CHAPTER 19

Walking on Broken Glass

APRIL 2019 – JULY 2019

Glimpses of hope materialize in the most abstract of ways: the heart-shaped cloud that appears out of nowhere during my darkest thoughts, the branches of the maple tree that create a cross, the cardinal that stares at me through the window for hours.

These gentle nudges from the universe interrupt the negative feedback loop of my mind, transporting me to a different place free from the harsh internal dialogue, and peace momentarily descends upon me. The slightest shift happens, a miniscule—almost undetectable—change in consciousness, the tiniest blip on a radar screen that disappears as suddenly as it appeared, makes me wonder if these brief moments of stillness and tranquility are an illusion. Focusing on these small signs, I say a silent *thank you* to a higher power and sit with myself and focus on the present moment, even if only for a minute. This is the work of creating new pathways in my brain. I can feel it.

Yet darkness is always luring me back under its cloak like an illicit activity. My mind tilts again; thoughts of positivity and better days ahead give way to a state of feverish chaos, frequent heart palpitations, a dull throbbing in my left temple, and hyperactivity, a Vegas slot machine at the mercy of a gambling addict.

I frantically clean the house to a sparkling shine, use a toothpick to reach the tiniest crumbs from the stove, self-clean the oven so much that the thermal fuse blows, move furniture to ensure every inch of carpet has been properly vacuumed, fold and refold laundry when it is not evenly creased, organize each junk drawer down to the last paper clip. I go through an entire box of dusting cloths, wipe each blind so not a speck of dust remains, and unscrew every light fixture, washing them in warm soapy water. Opening the kitchen cabinet containing the coffee mugs makes me panic, and I absolutely—*at this very minute*—must take everything out and purge all the mugs we no longer use because it is completely unacceptable to have an overflowing coffee mug cabinet. Or a disheveled silverware drawer.

The kids' play table has markers and stickers strewn about and is covered in coloring books, dried paint, and gummy residue from glue sticks gone astray. Dull tips of the bright Crayolas littering the floor enrage me and compel me to run to the store *right now* to buy a crayon sharpener. For the next few hours, sharpening the peeling, colorful tips becomes my sole priority. I push the waxy crayons in with reckless abandon, then get so angry when the sharpener jams up that I want to hurl it against the wall. I am fixated as though possessed, like my life depends on every crayon being perfectly pointy. Nolan picks up his sisters across the street at school because I refuse to leave my crayon-sharpening post.

It is only when letters start melding together that I admit something is seriously amiss. As I'm emailing a colleague, the words on the page scramble in front of my eyes, jump-roping across each other like double Dutch, to form incomprehensible gibberish like a word jumble. I type, "Thank wou," gaze intently at it, and convince myself that the W is a Y. I innately know that something is wrong but I'm unable to identify the exact culprit. When comprehension sets in, I call Dr. Nick and head to the lab for another round of bloodwork and testing.

The results are startling. My thyroid levels and antibodies are off the charts—almost 4,000 percent higher than normal range. Since the past few months have been spent detoxing heavy metals from my body, Dr. Nick concludes that I am in the middle of a thyroid storm, a rare condition that can cause cardiac arrest in severe cases.

Ever patient and calm as usual, he reassures me that the thyroid can go a bit haywire as heavy metals remove themselves from the deepest recesses of my cells. His advice is to stick to my protocol and stay the course—my body will rebalance itself—then get retested again in three months. I long to hear an uptick of concern in his voice, but instead his unworried response does little to placate the panic in my chest.

We hang up after several minutes, and I strongly question my decisions and his guidance, all our work together over the past 12 months, the natural healing techniques and supplements. Did I take the right path? My thoughts spiral like a tumbleweed in a desert storm. Would I have been better off with the traditional route of high-dose antibiotics for years instead? Should I have tried controversial stem cell therapy? Could my body innately heal itself on nature and instinct alone, without the help of synthetic manmade drugs? Am I truly going to survive this?

There is only one answer. Trusting my gut, I keep going. My anger fuels me forward in my determination to try anything left in natural healing to reclaim and take back control of my body. I research everything about chronic Lyme disease and thyroid storms and sample a variety of peculiar techniques that are not medically approved but have worked for someone, somewhere. I throw caution to the wind and use all available options that can potentially help.

I stumble upon Anthony William, the Medical Medium, a chronic illness expert who offers health advice based on communication with the spirit world. His cultlike following and reviews are extraordinary, and Amazon delivers several of his books to my doorstep the next morning. Devouring the lengthy tomes in a matter of days, I adjust my already restricted diet even more, and I solely consume foods he recommends are healing for thyroid and autoimmune conditions: bananas, cucumbers, kale, broccoli, cauliflower, arugula, garlic cloves. Committing to a nine-day raw fruit and vegetable cleanse causes major mood swings and more irritability. I hate every minute of it, but I stick to it, following the instructions down to every last detail and making no deviations. I even leave my beloved shaker of salt untouched for the full 216 hours.

The real kicker of this cleanse is the heavy metal detox smoothie first thing in the morning. Bananas, wild blueberries, one juiced orange, coconut water—all this sounds delicious by itself. Add in cilantro, spirulina (a blue-green algae), barley grass juice extract, and Atlantic dulse flakes (a type of seaweed), and the smell alone is enough to make me gag. Plugging my nose and closing my eyes, I force myself to choke it down. I tell myself that *this* will remove all the heavy metals from my body, nourish my cells, calm the storm raging within.

Anthony William has an entire book dedicated solely to the benefits of celery juice, so I purchase a juicer and clear out the organic celery section at the grocery store. He claims celery juice is a powerful healing remedy and consuming it on an empty stomach every morning can assist with healing from all kinds of acute and chronic illnesses. Eating celery does not have the same effect as juicing, which removes the pulp and allows the concentrated salts to increase bile production, rebuild hydrochloric stomach acid, and restore the central nervous system by flushing out toxins and poisons from the liver and other organs.

The juicer roars to life every morning. It gets stuck when my impatient hands shove too many stalks of celery into the top opening, forcing me to empty the fluffy green pulp into the garbage before continuing. I juice an entire bunch, sometimes two, each day, then greedily drink in the sixteen ounces of chartreuse saltiness. I start to crave the taste of it before my coffee, and I adjust the timing of my supplement schedule so it does not interfere with my new morning routine. Instead of gin and juice, I'm sippin' on celery juice.

My body responds instantaneously; horrific stomach pain jolts me out of bed the first night and ferocious vomiting leaves me sleeping on the bathroom floor, inches from the toilet bowl. Spasms flood my lower back but pale in comparison to the strong cramping in my uterus. Hours later I eliminate the grossest parasite yet—an otherworldly creature, ropelike and slimy, that looks like it came from the depths of the ocean. Although disgusted at the vileness of this situation and discouraged by the knowledge that there can still be parasites in me after more than a year of killing them off, I instantly feel better physically and mentally as soon as it is out of me.

The celery juice and rotating antiparasitics work in tandem, and the parasites now come out in droves. I feel them as they die, clinging to the lining of my stomach wall with their hooks and suckers before finally admitting defeat and succumbing to the mounting strength and offense of my intestinal tract. I drink gallons of organic bone broth, which is high in protein and can help with gut health. The gelatin in it is supposedly able to seal holes in the intestines and reduce overall inflammation.

I buy a "zapper," a small plastic rectangular box that runs on a 9-volt battery. There are two thin copper discs on the exterior of the box to place against my skin. When you turn the battery on, this contraption pulses at a frequency range of 14 to 16 Hertz, which produces a positive-offset wave form. Are you following this? Me neither. But several people in the Lyme community swear by it, so I give it a shot. I hold the zapper to my moistened lips and feel a small electrical current, satisfied that it actually does something and is not a complete hoax.

The frequency it emits supposedly kills parasites and viruses and encourages the growth of good bacteria, so I add this to my daily arsenal. The copper discs start to tingle and zing my skin after an hour, so I move it from the right side of my waistband to the left side. I put it inside my bra, tape it to my inner thigh, and sleep with it against the sole of my foot. I cannot tell if it does anything other than leave dark circle imprints that tattoo my body for days.

Weekly visits to the chiropractor adjust the kinks in my neck and stimulate my swollen, stagnant lymph nodes to open and drain the sludge out of my body. Foot reflexology massages are pleasant but produce no noticeable difference. A professional colonic is mortifying; coffee enemas in the privacy of my own bathroom are much preferred and more effective. The quiet stillness of a Himalayan salt room is peaceful, yet breathing in air filled with salt particles that are supposed to boost the immune system feels no different than breathing in air outside.

Dr. Cass Ingram, a nutritional physician and natural medicine pioneer, healed himself of a life-threatening case of chronic Lyme disease using wild medicinal spice extracts, the most prominent and potent one being oil of oregano. He has since written many books on natural healing and happens to be lecturing at a local hotel, so I arrive early, sit eagerly in the first row like a teacher's pet, and hang in rapt attention on his words as if they are gold.

His intensity matches his wild hair and bushy eyebrows, the passion in his voice so loud he is nearly yelling. The audience hoots and hollers in agreement like the shouted "Amen" of a worshipper in Sunday church.

Books and products are available for purchase, and I am suckered in like I'm watching a late-night infomercial. I'm intoxicated by the promise of a cure and suffocated by the overwhelming aroma of oregano. I buy it all—bottles of liquid oregano, spruce, and pine, cinnamon liquid mixed with oregano that masks the bitter taste for the kids, and a tub of oregano and spruce cream that I slather on every day, the pungent paste sinking into my arms and helping my cells battle off the offenders. I do not care that I smell like a walking spice rack.

My cognitive function improves.

My energy levels slowly increase.

I am certain my body is physically healing from the inside out.

I go in for blood work again, and the difference is astounding. Although my levels are still off the charts, they are now only 1,500 percent higher instead of the 4,000 percent from a few months ago. Unsure which remedy is responsible, I continue with all of them, knowing they all contributed to better health in some way or form. I am determined to keep going, ferocious in fact.

I have enough energy to occasionally attend hot yoga, where I am embarrassed by the litter box stench of my sweat but happy for the gentle movement of my body and the recession of anxiety and panic that allows me to leave the house.

While slower than usual, I walk a mile around our block with our faithful pit bull, Hailey, and I enjoy our time together outside in nature. Blue jays appear overhead, their shrill jeers and squawks like a young child desperate for attention. "Look at me!" My eyes are drawn skyward, and I watch their rambunctious flight path as they follow us like sheep. The blue jay symbolizes intuition and spiritual energy, and spirit guides use them to show you that you are on the right track in life.

I don't believe in coincidences.

CHAPTER 20

In Sickness and In Health

AUGUST 2020

Dan was supportive in my pursuit of healing. He attended most coaching calls with Dr. Nick alongside me and changed his diet and tried new recipes to accommodate the dwindling list of foods that were safe for me to eat. His interest slowly waned as time ticked by—the initial excitement tempered as each passing month resulted in only incremental improvements. Both of us were disappointed that recovery was taking so long, and he was frustrated by the snaillike pace of the progress I was making.

When we spoke our wedding vows to each other years ago, we were in the prime of life. We were blissfully naïve that sickness would become such a large part of our marriage. The strain of chronic illness tiptoed delicately in, glided sneakily into our everyday routine, discreet and inconspicuous until it became such an unignorable third wheel that our marriage fractured, with tiny fissures growing as large as my daily supplement count. The solid foundation we created over time was crumbling into burgeoning resentment, and I began to question if we were strong enough to get through this.

I was no longer the flirtatious and playful vixen Dan married or the wife who lobbed back verbal quips as quickly as he dished them out. My bygone quick wit was lost in the haziness of my misfiring brain. Our once lighthearted banter was now relegated to talk of my supplement and nap schedules, the dinner menu, calendar management, and the upcoming activities our children needed to attend.

The brunt of household and child-rearing obligations fell on Dan's shoulders when Lyme disease rendered me useless and confined me to my bed for days at a time, unable to do anything more than sleep. The previously balanced roles of husband and wife shifted to those of caretaker and patient, the scales tipping and creating an unequal division of responsibilities with Dan compensating largely for my lack. His time and patience were already stretched thin from a demanding career, and our relationship became a pressure cooker waiting to explode. Our communication was taut, a precarious tightrope that could break with one wrong word, one accusatory sideways glance, one overly loud agitated sigh.

I was angry at the work commitments he still expected me to show up to, the dinners and the parties, the family gatherings we continued to host. We have always been the "yes" couple.

"Yes, we'd love to come to your pool party even though I have to sleep on your couch all day." "Yes, we'd be happy to host at our house yet again." "Yes, even though I just did a coffee enema and pulled parasites out of my ass, I can still make the office tailgate."

Our initial attempt at dealing with the shifting power dynamics in our marriage was to ignore it. This strategy backfired as the dust bunnies of pain we brushed under the rug grew larger each week.

Equating sickness with weakness, a trait I never want to be associated with, I kept the charade going. I continued to present a false sense of self in front of others. Dan was the only other person who truly shared the full burden of my disease. The strength imbued into me after Mom died made frailty a trigger for me, so I covered up and downplayed my illness in public to avoid being seen as weak.

I smiled at the right times, laughed gauchely at terribly inappropriate jokes, asked questions about kids and families, told everyone I was feeling better and not to worry. And then when the party was over, our appearance there complete, I stewed silently in the car on the way home, offended that I'd had to leave the house to attend a function where no one would truly miss my presence anyway.

Stomping angrily up the stairs to the bedroom, I would slam the door and go directly to bed, pulling up the covers so aggressively that the sheet would come untucked from the bottom of the mattress. Dan would enter moments later, open dresser drawers forcefully, brush his teeth and climb into bed, and always be the first to initiate any difficult conversation. We spun around and around, repeatedly said the same words to each other, and hoped that this time our conversation would somehow yield a different outcome.

I would lie there in awkward silence until Dan exasperatedly kicked off our circular argument. "I don't understand what's going on. How can you be so happy around others and then the second we're alone, you turn into someone else? You're not the person you used to be."

I sighed. "You're right. I'm not. I used to love going out, but now I feel forced to go to events even when I feel terrible. I can't continue to do this. It's only setting me back."

"It's not just that—you enjoy being around others more than me. We barely talk anymore, and when we do, you speak in two-word sentences. I work so hard to provide for our family, do the grocery shopping, cook dinner, take care of the kids so you can rest, but it's never appreciated and not enough for you."

"That's not true. I appreciate everything you do and your support of me."

"Well, it doesn't seem like it. You show love to the kids but not me. You treat me with apathy, and I want you to respect and love me like you used to."

"I *do* love you, but I don't know what you want from me or what more I can give right now. I'm not pretending to be sick. I'm pretending to be well. *We* need to stop pretending that I can do everything I used to."

"Are you pretending to still love me?"

That stung. The conversation was over, both of us turning off our bedside lamps and turning our backs to each other in exasperation. I digested his words as the accuracy of them sunk in. My sole priority was raising our children and keeping myself alive as our marriage took a backseat. Our scripted arguments had the same snippy back and forth, the "I don't feel good/you don't appreciate me" ringing in our ears long after they were over. Neither of us knew how to get off our dysfunctional carousel ride that spun us around in dizzying circles. As the distance between us grew wider, we turned to Islena for help with couples coaching calls.

Islena listened intently, nodded along, and heard both of us out—my frustration at being expected to live life as usual, portraying a pretense of health, and Dan feeling underappreciated and unloved with my lack of attention to him.

She weighed in with her sage advice: "The purpose of marriage is not to make you happy—it's for personal development. Conflict and communication breakdown are just a difference in priorities at that moment. Sarah, your priority is on healing. Dan, your priority is on family, communication, and stability. Neither of you is wrong for your priorities."

I justified my point of view. "Dan seems annoyed when I have particularly bad days—like he is jealous of my illness, as though I intentionally choose to be sick and miss family dinners and bedtime prayers. When I need to rest, his whole demeanor changes."

I thought about the slight flare of anger that erupted in his speckled blue eyes, the limp hugs we gave each other, the tightening of his lips and the barely-there pecks on the cheek. I remembered night after night of my nearly imperceptible shift away from him in bed to avoid any form of intimacy, my desire nonexistent. I no longer cared about meeting his basic manly needs, even knowing full well his love language was physical touch and affection. He held me hostage with unspoken words of affirmation, and I held him hostage with celibacy.

Dan clarified. "I walk in the door after a long day and Sarah doesn't greet me. No hug, no kiss like she used to. She doesn't want to engage. She's despondent and goes to bed as soon as I get home."

The three of us were quiet until Islena broke the silence. "In every relationship you will experience rejection, not because you or your partner are wrong, but because they are unable to be who you want them to be in that moment. You are in a period of significant change, individually and as a couple, and your communication style needs to adapt to this. You are both stuck in the comfort zone of how your marriage was prior to Sarah getting sick. Staying in that zone can be a toxic place, as you are experiencing with your communication breakdowns. Your marriage is not the same anymore and you need to figure out—together—how to create a new normal that works for you, a place where you both feel seen and heard."

I asked, "And how exactly do we do that?"

"I'd like you to construct a mission statement for your marriage. It doesn't have to be fancy, but you should cocreate this together, take turns writing sentences about what you need from each other, what you want your marriage to look like, how you will overcome conflict in the future. You should update this as your marriage evolves and your needs change."

I cringed as she continued. "Think of this as a safe environment to express yourself, to be open and honest with no fear of judgment or rejection. The more you are aware of what your partner needs, the better you can communicate effectively with each other. Our calls together are just the beginning. The true hard work happens during the in-between times, the small daily changes you make, the effort you put in to understanding each other."

Dan and I sat on the couch together and took turns awkwardly writing with a red felt-tip pen. We wrote about building a solid foundation for our children, having passion and fun in all that we do, letting go of past baggage, addressing conflict in the moment, creating boundaries that work for our family, and holding hands in our rocking chairs when we are old and gray.

We taped it to our bathroom mirror and read it morning and night as we brushed our teeth, a bright-red reminder of what we wanted our marriage to be, what we needed from each other, how we could be better partners. On the brink of a more meaningful, deeper relationship, we were committed to having a marriage that survived chronic illness.

It was a messy work in progress as we stumbled through arguments and tried to hold space for each other amid the discomfort when I would rather shut down and ice him out with the silent treatment. My need to rest was still there, but during our quiet moments together, I tried to stay present. I told Dan how much I appreciated and loved him, inquired about his day, asked if there was anything I could do for him.

As our marriage got stronger through increased dialogue, Dan felt more open to share his perspective with me. We were in a place where he could finally let out the anger, sadness, and frustration he had kept bottled up. He knew that we were now solid enough to have the raw, difficult conversations.

Since healing became my priority, everything else fell to the wayside. Dan admitted this was necessary to a degree, and the pain in his voice was clearly evident as he described the impact of my illness on him, how I inadvertently invalidated his feelings and perspective. How my words, or lack thereof, cut him deep, how he misinterpreted my sole focus on healing as apathy, lost in translation like a game of telephone in middle school.

We have intimate conversations in real time now with more transparency and authenticity. We no longer walk on eggshells. We occasionally get furious with each other, but now we sit with the anger together until it passes. We do our best to let go of bitter missteps and stale arguments long past. We try even when we don't feel like it, reading our marriage statement together through gritted teeth after particularly maddening spats until we laugh.

The "yes" mentality we adhered to before is not sustainable now that Lyme disease has stolen the show and taken center stage. Our work commitments overlap with social commitments, and while I find cancelling at the last minute to be tasteless and rude in most circumstances, my health and the well-being of our marriage takes precedence. I shed my worry about others' opinions and no longer feel guilty for staying home and resting while Dan flies solo to events that I had previously committed to. We recognize that it is perfectly acceptable to show up as individuals instead of as a couple when necessary. We discuss boundaries and say "no" to things that do not truly bring us joy. We are more discerning about where and who we spend our time and energy with.

We renew our vows after our ten-year wedding anniversary in the exact same spot we got married. Surrounded by our family, our oldest child, Nolan, officiates a brief ceremony and the younger two, Everly and Addy, each do a reading before we all pour different colors of sand into a glass frame. I tear up at the beauty around us and see the raw emotion in Dan's eyes. Our marriage is that much stronger now from all the good and bad combined.

It is hard to forget pain, but even more difficult to remember happiness. The good times don't leave a scar, no shiny silvery puckered reminder of the pain endured. I want to remember every moment of our ceremony today, the vows we speak to each other, the sun shining on us and our family. This ceremony represents all our hard work, everything we have overcome, our willingness to rebuild our marriage and rediscover who we are after all of this and to create better versions of ourselves—together—till death do us part.

CHAPTER 21

This Is 40

AUGUST 2019

I joyfully wave goodbye to 39 with my middle finger high. I am more than ready to put the last few years firmly in the rearview mirror. Dan and I celebrate my milestone 40th birthday at Mii Amo, a wellness spa in Sedona, Arizona, that inspires guests to focus on well-being, to journey within themselves and find connection with nature and their surroundings. With only 16 guest rooms, it is a secluded resort hideaway that provides solitude and privacy for those who seek it.

Truth be told, I did not think I would live to see 40, so I want this birthday to be extra special, to signify the start of a new decade of health and wellness. I chose Sedona for the magic of the energy vortexes that are concentrated in its geography. An energy vortex is a location in nature where the earth's energy is amplified, where it flows in a spiraling, swirling motion, creating a powerful and dynamic force. Vortex sites are considered conduits for spiritual connection—to nature, the divine, or one's inner self—and are known to reduce stress and anxiety and provide clarity, emotional healing, and personal empowerment.

Mii Amo is in the heart of Boynton Canyon, a famous energy vortex associated with magnetic energy, believed to enhance meditation, inner exploration, spirituality, and a deeper sense of self. My heart races with excitement as we drive our Jeep over the dusty roads, stirring up red powder and earth that covers the car behind us like a blanket.

The red rocks and exposed outcroppings of the landscape dwarf all else. I crane my neck at an almost 90-degree angle to see the sky and clouds beyond the high rust-colored plateaus, the brightness of the turquoise blue highlighting the deep crimson of the cliffs and crevices formed from years of erosion and shifting tectonic plates. Junipers and towering pines are scattered throughout, and soaring rock spires and unique color formations showcase millions of years of oxidation and evolution.

Upon our arrival at the gated spa, a personal attendant greets us with juniper-beaded necklaces handmade by the local Yavapai Apache tribe. She bows her head and says, "*Yah-na-say*," which means "You are welcome here." A charm of hummingbirds flits about the courtyard trees, the peaceful quiet allowing us to hear the frantic flapping of their wings, as if we're surrounded by hundreds of lazy bumblebees. These tiny creatures look like they're treading water midair as their forked tongues flick in and out tasting the sweet nectar of the flowers and lapping up the sugar water.

After checking into our casita, replete with fireplace and heated bathroom floors, we head to the Crystal Grotto, a circular space with a red earthen floor and an arched ceiling. A small skylight allows the sun and the moon to beam down into the center, illuminating the petrified wood, soothing fountain, and quartz crystal. An employee named Wendy leads the communal welcome ritual, where we meet several of the staff as well as other guests who checked in today and are beginning their journeys.

We go around the circle as guests introduce themselves and tell the group why they are here and what they hope to gain from this experience. Several women are there for a girls' trip, an older couple is celebrating their 30th wedding anniversary, there's a mother-and-daughter duo, and a few solo travelers who say their names but nothing else. When it's my turn, I barely get my name out before bursting into uncontrollable tears, then I tell these strangers through sniffles and hiccups that my intention is to heal the brokenness inside. Nods of support encircle me, and several of the others' eyes water in understanding. Dan squeezes my hand tightly.

Exiting the Crystal Grotto, our group moves on to the Labyrinth Walk, a continuous circular path in the grass that twists and turns, eventually leading to the center. It's different from a maze in that there is only one way in and out. Labyrinths are a moving meditation tool that can unwind the mind and release behavioral patterns, allowing you to let go of burdens when you reach the center.

Wendy hands each of us a small leather pouch and instructs us to write our deepest intention on a piece of paper. She tells us to word our intention in the affirmative, that positivity resonates greater with our human spirits than negativity. On another piece of paper, we write what we want to let go of, what we have been carrying and are now ready to release.

There are so many intentions and things to relinquish, but I finally settle on the ones that are loudest. I firmly write on one piece of paper: *I am willing to receive God's help.* And on the other piece: *I surrender my physical and emotional sickness.*

We all place both pieces in our tan pouches and hang them around our necks, then our group lines up at the beginning of the labyrinth. Wendy waves a bundle of sage over us before we enter, and then we slowly start walking into the labyrinth. At the center, there is the option to drop our piece of paper with what we want to let go of into a bowl or to keep it in our pouch; I gladly drop mine into the bowl. Once everyone is done, Wendy transfers the slips of paper from the bowl into a large abalone shell. Then she lights a match, and we watch as the paper turns to ash. We stand that much taller as the smoke of our burdens floats away on the warm breeze.

The services Dan and I have chosen over the course of our four-day journey are a mixture of massage, body treatments, meditations, and energy work, including intuitive readings and past-life regression. Hiking the short Boynton Canyon Trail in the mornings before our first service of the day is tiring, but I am ecstatic to have enough energy to exercise again. A flute player named Robert sits atop Warrior Rock and shouts out, "This song is for healing!" The sound makes me stop in my tracks to sit on the earth and listen to the haunting melody. Lizards and deer peer out behind lone trees and boulders in curiosity.

My facial and body treatments are decadently indulgent, and afterward I linger at the large panes of glass in the treatment room that provide sweeping views of the canyon. The sheer size and immensity of this geographical wonder remind me of the insignificance of most of the worries that plague me, the enormity of this sacred ground a stark reminder that we are temporary inhabitants of this beautiful earth that will still be here long after we are.

Rain thrashes the roof during my past-life regression, pounding in time with the drum that the practitioner gently beats and hums along to. The year 1922 flashes in my mind. Dan is by my side as I lie dying. He places a cool compress on my forehead as tendrils of gray hair frame my face, and I know that we are truly soulmates and have been together in a previous lifetime.

Dan connects deeply with his spirit animal, the wolf. He buys a gigantic wolf head statue and teases me by howling at the moon. A joint tarot card reading provides a clear picture of our life together and reveals that we are in a period of great transformation—individually and as a couple—and we should let it unfold naturally. Accept where we are right now, embrace the lessons, learn and grow from them, stop clinging to the past and let it go.

We chant together in the Crystal Grotto with two other guests who are classically trained opera singers. We laugh uncontrollably at the sound of our out-of-tune voices reverberating off the walls, mere karaoke singers in the presence of Beyoncé.

We reconvene for lunch each afternoon at the aptly named Hummingbird restaurant for fresh-pressed juices and nourishing smoothies before parting ways for our separate early-evening treatments. My private chakra meditation in the Crystal Grotto is overwhelming. Dressed only in my flowing robe, I sit awkwardly on the bench as the guide walks me into a meditative state. Tears flow from start to finish.

Afterward, the guide sits next to me and places her hands upon mine. "Let the tears come," she says. "They will heal your heart. You are already a part of God and he is everywhere—the air you breathe, the sounds you hear, the people you meet, your children's laugh, the ground you walk on. He is supporting you, healing you. He loves you. Do not be afraid anymore. You are supported and watched over."

During an intuitive massage, my masseuse, Andrea, speaks with me the entire time, explaining what sort of energy she senses, what messages she is picking up from the universe. She asks what traumatic loss I endured when I was a very young girl and feels that this had a profound impact on me. I get choked up, as I immediately know what she is referring to, and travel back in time to July 1985.

The six-passenger twin-engine Cessna 414 hit the ground hard and fast. My grandfather and uncle were coming home from a father-son fishing trip in Ontario when the pilot had a heart attack and lost consciousness. Flight control picked up a mayday call from Grandpa Hy and then the aircraft disappeared from the radar moments later, leaving no survivors among the twisted metal of the flaming wreckage.

My sixth birthday was in three weeks. Mom and I stood in Grammy's kitchen, adorned with red, white, and blue decorations to celebrate the Fourth of July in two days. They talked to each other in hushed voices while I played with the early birthday present Grandpa had given me before he left for his trip—a My Little Pony horse stable. Every detail of that moment is still etched into my mind. They went quiet and I saw them crying. I asked what was wrong and walked toward them, past the giant mint-green typewriter, past the Brinks alarm system that would always beep in the middle of the night, past the gold spray-painted SHIT sign that Grammy thought was hilarious.

Mom, knelt to my eye level and said with her voice quavering, "Sarah, Grandpa Hy and Uncle Dick died in a plane crash. They won't be coming home again, which is why we are so sad."

I peered into her watery eyes, saw the trembling of her hands, then turned my attention upward toward Grammy, who stood there shaking her head back and forth in disbelief, open-mouthed and whimpering. Unsure and not fully understanding the meaning or magnitude of these words, I laughed—a deep, resounding belly laugh that was completely inappropriate for the circumstances. This involuntary response was so unexpected, and I innately knew that it was wrong but I had no control over it. The guilt for reacting this way has stayed with me for years.

Describing this to Andrea, I question if this was the start of my emotional dysregulation, of not being able to feel emotions properly. She explains that this can be a common human response during traumatic events. As the mind tries to protect itself, the nervous system gets overwhelmed and goes into self-preservation mode. Expressions like this happen when strong emotions are present and there is excess energy, which comes out in a way that looks different from what we are feeling internally, i.e., laughing instead of crying.

Andrea asks if I have heard of my inner child. *Dammit, I thought Islena worked through all of this with me already.* Then she has me look at and talk to my five-year-old self and forgive her for laughing. She did nothing wrong. She was an innocent child unprepared to face such a huge loss at such a young age. I do as she says, sobbing as she continues to lightly massage me. I feel like I am staring directly into my youngest daughter's eyes as I console my younger self once again.

I am exhausted and mentally depleted once the massage is done, and Andrea guides me back to the serene lounge. She tells me that my aura is like a centuries-old tree—it gets stronger with each storm that makes its roots dig deeper into the ground. She cautions me to have patience, to find grace and compassion for all versions of myself, and to be gentle as I find my way back.

The last morning of our trip, I write furiously in a small red journal, a gift left by the housekeeping staff on my pillow alongside a dream catcher. I stretch my legs, content in my aloneness on the casita patio while Dan packs his suitcase, and write down details so I can dissect and remember them later. I am grateful for this opportunity, for the beautiful people here who are filled with such light and love, for this new sense of hope and renewal. This trip commemorates all the healing work of both my body and mind.

Wanting to soak up every ounce of the transformative energy of the canyon in our last moments here, I look up at the red rocks once more. A shock wave ripples through me as a hawk flies overhead. It screeches its high-pitched "keeeeee-arrrrr" as though it is talking directly to me, and I envision my brother, Mike, watching over and guiding me from above. I feel a strong presence, closer to a higher power than ever before. I understand that my journey is about accepting the present moment and embracing the transformation before me, that I can still show up for life and experience happiness even in the midst of illness.

CHAPTER 22

Rise Up

SEPTEMBER 2019 – DECEMBER 2019

Fall arrives the way all seasons do, slowly at first, with the leaves crisp under my feet, brittle and crunchy as the kids playfully throw them at each other during an animated game of tag. The bite of chilly air turns their noses and cheeks pink. The euphoria from Sedona is fading as quickly as the daylight does this time of year. Nature innately understands that now is a time to decelerate, rest, enjoy a slower pace. I long to be more like the trees—boldly shedding what no longer serves them, exposing themselves to the harshness of winter, letting the leaves of the past transform into vibrant red, orange, and gold memories. They are a reminder of how beautiful it is to let go.

Letting go has never been a strength of mine. Bitterness, anger, sadness, and grief toward those who have wronged or hurt me in the past, including myself, are imbued within my cells, as permanent a part of me as my own heartbeat. Rewiring my brain takes time and mental setbacks occur regularly. Holding on to stories of the past is hindering my spiritual growth and healing, and I long to free myself of the heavy baggage.

The smallest thing sets me off and triggers something from years ago—a song, smell, picture, color, words a stranger mutters in passing at the grocery store—and the downward spiral becomes so steep, the darkness so absolute, that I cannot find my way out. Depression extinguishes any sense of happiness I have experienced with my progress and health recovery in the last few months. My invisible scars are still raw and red. They pulsate and undulate with melancholy, proving the cliché that time heals all wounds a fallacy. How shattered does one have to be before they stop trying to put the pieces back together? How much more can there possibly be to heal?

Yo-yoing between happiness and despair within seconds, my uncontrollable mood swings scare me as I hover in a manic-depressive state. I lean against the wall of the garage. Blue sky and dazzling sunlight pierce my eyes as the girls ride their bikes with training wheels around the driveway. All I feel is despondent, longing for an end. I envision closing the garage door with my truck running and drifting off melodically into the ether.

I call my father in desperation, sugarcoating the sadness, and tell him about all the mental work and processing of grief that I have done but how it still doesn't seem to be enough to ease the pain. His concern is apparent, and he asks to come over. I politely decline, then he suggests that going back on Prozac may help. My shelves are lined with books about owning myself, my mind, my body; they are visual evidence of the one-sided mindset I have subscribed to that synthetic pills are the work of the devil himself. The thought of relying on a tiny little pill for the rest of my life to dictate my emotional well-being is insulting, but if the alternative is self-harm and suicidal ideation, then my ego and pride need to sit in the backseat and surrender to the beauty of manmade prescription drugs.

It is time to stop being a martyr for natural health. My pendulum had swung so wildly in one direction that I eschewed Western medicine entirely. Seeing my daughters' tangled blond hair billowing in the breeze, hearing their pure squeals of laughter and joy as their little legs pedal and pick up speed on the small downward slope, listening to my father's voice deep and serious in my ear, I realize that this is all that truly matters. I only have this day, this moment, this second, before it is gone, and I need to rise above. Rise above the pain, the past, the opinions of others, the hurt, the grief, the sickness, all of it. This is another chance to react differently, to create a new pattern, to let my determination continue to push me toward *all* possible healing tools.

I begrudgingly place a call to my primary care doctor, who I have not seen in several years, and make an appointment to discuss restarting Prozac. I surrender to healing no matter what it looks like or what form it comes in. I allow myself the grace to embrace the best of both alternative and conventional medicine. I am not a failure for accepting help with my mental health. Surrendering does not mean giving up—it is simply releasing the energy of struggle and making the conscious decision to heal instead of fight.

Knowing it will take some time before the effects of the happy pills kick in, I take the same approach I did during the thyroid storm. I make myself a guinea pig, try everything possible, and muscle through as long as necessary until something clicks.

Islena and Dr. Nick tout the benefits of meditation every time we speak, but it has never truly worked for me. My mind runs unchaperoned and wild as a stallion. I attend a class at a community center on how to meditate where I meet other people from all walks of life, and I relate to their similar sentiments of being unable to quiet the incessant chatter in their brains. We listen intently to the instructor as we sit crisscross applesauce on the floor if our knees allow or with legs stretched in front for those with achy joints, our derrieres propped up by a pillowy bolster. My legs are pretzeled beneath me as sounds of deep breathing fill the room, loudly at first and then quieting in hushed synchronization. Although my mind wanders, awareness sets in—the beating of my heart, the kaleidoscope shapes that appear behind closed eyelids, the rank smell of the woman next to me—before everything fades away and my sole focus becomes my breath.

It doesn't last long as my attention turns to my now fully asleep legs, which I slowly unfurl as quietly as possible, pins and needles pricking from hip to ankle. Cracking open my eyes, I am bored, restless. I wonder how much longer we are going to do this. Surely it has been at least twenty minutes by now. Glancing at the clock on the wall, I see only six minutes have passed, so I find a different position and try again. I focus on my breath for slightly longer than before and get lost in the silence. When the instructor tells us to open our eyes, I feel relaxed and tired. I download a meditation app on my phone and commit to meditating for a minimum of ten minutes each day.

I fall asleep every time, frustrated that I cannot do it "correctly," but I keep practicing. Three weeks later, I have my first true glimpse of the joy of meditation when my mind clears fully and I can just *be*, simply allow my breath and the here and now to be enough.

The soothing voice of the guided meditations are so calming that I still fall asleep but I awaken rejuvenated, in a better frame of mind than when I began. Meditation becomes an outlet for my emotional well-being, a regular practice in my daily routine. It keeps me grounded and present, one more small tool in my arsenal of re-regulating my dysfunctional nervous system. I enjoy it so much that I attend a full-day silent meditation retreat in a freezing-cold room. I eat lunch in silence, mindful of every bite, watch a solitary leaf fall to the snow-covered ground, and nod off and fall asleep on a stranger's shoulder during the group meditations.

A friend who is going through her own personal growth and transformation process had a profound experience with a reiki practitioner named Brenda, so I take her advice and schedule an appointment. Reiki comes from the Japanese words *rei*, meaning universal, and *ki*, which refers to a flow of life force energy. Practitioners place their hands on or near their client's body to help release and balance their energy fields, staying in one place for a few minutes before moving to a different part of the body.

Driving to Brenda's studio, a memory from years ago flashes through my mind when a woman at the gym told me she was a reiki master, causing me to judge her harshly and label her a wacko. The tables have turned, and I now tsk at my younger self for being so critical and narrow-minded. The quaint studio is bathed in taupe tones and fake candlelight, and I suddenly have a craving for hot chocolate as Brenda greets me. She's blonde-haired and blue-eyed and bears a striking resemblance to the Swiss Miss woman, as though she has just returned from yodeling in the Alps with her flock of sheep.

Fully clothed, I lie down on the massage table and close my eyes, inhale deeply, and try to remain present. The light pressure Brenda applies to my feet, knees, and legs is comfortable, the tension in my body slowly melting away. When she places her hands on my hips, a warmth rises within, and the intensity is so hot it borders on uncomfortable. Opening my eyes and gazing down at my hips, I expect to see heating pads, but it is just her two hands gently resting there. I breathe through the warmth and tell myself it's just an illusion. Angel wings appear in my mind's eye and a light breeze whispers across the room.

Once our session is over, Brenda mentions that every now and then when working on a client, a cool breeze will pass by her face, which happened several times when she was working on my hips. I tell her I assumed the air conditioner was turning on.

"Sarah, those were angels. They are working on you as well."

On my way out, there are advertisements for float therapy and other psychic healers, so I snag business cards for each one. Strongly sensing that all these things are somehow connected, that each therapy or session I try points my body and mind toward balance, shows me the right next step, I follow the subtle clues like I'm on a scavenger hunt and tune into my intuition and perhaps the divine intervention that is occurring right before my eyes.

My tortured soul still cries out for help, and a shamanic mediumship session with Jen at The Soul Source feels like the next right step. Jen only asks for my first name when I book the appointment and gives me directions to her private home and studio. The familiar fall sky is gray and dull on my drive there. Dark clouds hang like leaden balloons and block out the sun, which has been a stranger for weeks now.

Barking dogs greet me as I gingerly push open the front door, take my shoes off, and wait in the tiny vestibule that smells like freshly burned sage. Jen calls out from the kitchen and invites me to enter fully.

She guides me through the living room into her office at the end of the narrow hallway. She describes her practice and how she lights a fire outside for every client before the initial meeting. She tells me that the one she lit for me kept burning out, like all the joy has been extinguished from my life.

Clamming up when she asks what my goal is for our time together, I nervously spit out, "I'm not entirely sure what it is I'm looking for."

Nodding in understanding, she closes her eyes and takes a deep breath in. "Let's see what comes through." Moments later, her eyes fly open. "Are your parents divorced, or do you have two separate sets of parents?"

"Nope."

"Hmmm. There are four distinct family units stepping forward, but two are sticking closer to the wall, like they are afraid to come closer. Was there a falling out in the family?"

"Not that I'm aware of. I was adopted and—"

"*Aha!* That makes sense. Your biological family are the ones in the back. They are quieter but watching over you nonetheless as you are still part of them."

"Wow, I never met any biological relatives, and I don't know anything about them."

"It doesn't matter. Familial ties transcend space and time. There are two other females very close to you, almost jostling for position. I'm picking up a strong grandmotherly energy and she is right next to you. The image she shows me is of you as a child in a frilly red dress, strawberry-blonde hair, full of joy and laughter. She is wondering where that girl went."

Chuckling, I respond. "That sounds like Grammy. We had a special bond, and I was closer to her than to my mother."

"Her love and adoration for you is clear. Your mother is behind her. Her energy is one of emotional unavailability but also of overwhelming love. She carried a tremendous amount of guilt about leaving so much unfinished and unspoken."

Tears stream down my face.

"Sarah, I know this is difficult for you to hear, but your mom wants you to stop carrying her burden. She has already released this and is happy on the other side. You are the only one still suffering here. It's time to let go of the anger and grief. She wants you to move on, experience and enjoy the beauty of this world, receive and allow gratitude into your life. Her death does not define you. Whatever you are going through right now does not define you."

I purse my mouth into a large O as I try to figure out how to respond to this. I am speechless, astonished that this woman knows this, senses this, hears this. I have told her nothing about my life other than my first name, and unlike prior people claiming they have clairvoyant powers, she clearly has a gift of communicating with the spirit world.

Jen continues. "I smell cigarette smoke. There is a young male here who keeps stepping forward and then back, hesitant because he's unsure if you want to hear from him. His passing was tragic, sudden, and unexpected. I'm hearing a nickname...hang on...it starts with an S—Sully?"

"Oh. My. God. That's my brother Mike. We all called him Sully. I can't believe you just said that."

"He has quite the personality. He watches over your daughters, but especially your youngest. He wants you to let go of your guilt. He lived the life he was destined to, and he wants you to remember all the silly times you had together, to remember the laughter."

Jen passes along several messages from other relatives, comforting words I was not expecting to hear, words that provide solace and peace, affirmation that even though my loved ones are no longer here physically, they are still with me in spirit.

I am ready to let go of my grief without letting go of my loved ones. I am ready to embrace their memories in a healing way rather than a traumatic one. As our session wraps up, I feel grateful for this intimate violation of my innermost demons, a violation I welcome and embrace.

Peace washes over me, and for the first time since their deaths, I feel like I can finally close this chapter of grief. Letting go is not only enabling me to embrace all methods of physical healing but also is becoming a driving force for my emotional healing. It is time to stop letting the stories of my past dictate my future. It is time to find my joy.

CHAPTER 23

When I Come Around

JANUARY 2020 – MARCH 2020

It is an unseasonably warm day for this time of year, and rivers of melting ice flow through the gym parking lot with nowhere to go as sewer grates get clogged with the dirty debris of winter. People slip and slide on their way to the entrance, unsure if the ground they step on is black ice or just water. I tiptoe cautiously to the large glass doors and nervously enter the fitness facility like it's the first day of a new school. My palms are sweaty with anticipation and trepidation is coursing through my veins. Nothing has changed yet everything feels foreign. Being back here, in this pre-sickness environment that I spent so much time in, is triggering; it reminds me of how much energy I once had and how drastically different my life was a few short years ago.

The lingering symptoms of the thyroid storm wane and diminish almost entirely, and my cells are physically healing from the inside out. I am not fully recovered yet. I am still plagued by sporadic flare-ups of symptoms, but I feel well enough to remove the medical hold on my gym membership and activate it again.

Familiar faces and old friends greet me warmly. They embrace me in hugs and exclamations of "I'm so glad you're feeling better" and "It's so nice to have you back!" I recoil from their touch like it's a hot flame. I'm rigid as a board as their arms encircle me. They are eager to pick up right where we left off two years ago as though nothing has happened, as if they did not completely forget about me once I got sick, as if our friendship mattered. I am resentful that their lives are still the same. Anger bubbles up, and I respond with a curt "Thank you" before abruptly walking down the stairwell to the pool, where the only dialogue I must engage in is internal.

The lanes are longer than I remember—they must have doubled in size since my last swim—and my once-rapid laps are now lethargic and slow. My shoulders and arms burn with fatigue after only five minutes, and I hop out, dry off with the scratchy too-small gym towel, change in the locker room, and head upstairs to catch the second half of spin class. A stranger has claimed my favorite spin bike, so I hop on a rickety one in the back row with squeaky pedals. I feel out of place in a room that used to feel like home. I cycle at my own sloth-like pace and clip out immediately after class to avoid any small talk.

Before I shower off, I indulge in the welcome treat of the small sauna, a warm refuge to sweat out toxins and ease the pain in my joints. I pop my headphones in and listen to calming meditations with positive subliminal messages, turning the volume up to drown out the gossip of the crochety old ladies. I keep my eyes firmly closed, my nonverbals alerting others that I have no interest in conversing.

These quiet moments of introspective self-reflection are eye-opening and liberating. Sitting in the same spot that I used to in what seems like ages ago, memories flood back of the raucous laughter of the other gym moms and myself as we shared stories of diaper blowouts, tantrums, sleepless nights covered in spit-up, and mountains of spilled goldfish in the Costco checkout line. Other than the cackling grannies in the corner, the sauna is quieter today, just me and my thoughts, and some of the blame for the dissolution of friendships shifts to me. I recall the text messages I left unanswered, the invitations I turned down time and again, the phone calls I sent straight to voicemail, and the abrupt change in my attitude with no further explanation.

I have spent a great deal of time these past few years being angry at others—focusing on their faults, how they wronged me and were not there when I needed them most, how they questioned my health because I didn't look sick on the outside. I have completely discounted how my lack of engagement and reclusive tendencies played a role in the fading of friendships. Accountability now dawns on me like a new day, bathing me in rays of guilt, and I recognize that perhaps the stories of abandonment and estrangement I told myself existed only in the fictional abyss of my own mind.

I ponder this and pride myself on this elevated level of emotional awareness and clarity that allows me to see a discernable change in my thought pattern. The difference now is understanding. I now understand that it is acceptable to embrace my shortcomings and accept fault for things I have done wrong. I understand that the only one truly responsible for my self-worth, my emotional and physical health is me. It strikes me as ironic that chronic Lyme disease may be both the best and worst thing that I have had to overcome. It has changed every ounce of me physically and mentally, but I am beginning to understand that the strongest people are borne out of the darkest times. I release some of my anger and bless the splintered friendships.

I have a follow-up appointment with Nicole, the holistic wellness nurse practitioner, for another round of biomeridian testing. The computer spits out its sonar-sounding bleeps and whistles, but with less frequency than my last round of testing. While my immune system is definitively stronger, Lyme bacteria is very much present in my body.

Seeing my discouragement, Nicole reassures me. "Your body has shifted tremendously. It is a positive thing that the Lyme bacteria are showing up so strong right now. It's not buried deep within your cells in hiding or concealed by biofilm anymore. It's active, and now is the perfect time to eradicate it completely."

"I thought that's what I've been doing these past two years!"

Nicole chuckles. "Sarah, you were riddled with so many other tick-borne diseases, coinfections, parasites, and gut infections that needed to be addressed first. Now that you have cleared these out and boosted your immune system, you are strong enough to go after the last—and most formidable—adversary, which is the Lyme bacteria."

"OK, let's do it. I'm ready to get rid of this once and for all."

"These next three months are going to be intense. You have dealt with so much already, and I know you can handle this. I hate saying it, but you will likely have Herxheimer reactions, where you feel worse for a few weeks before you feel better. Know that this is normal and part of the process. Hang in there and it will pass. Let's schedule your next follow-up appointment for three months from now."

I leave her office feeling frustrated but encouraged, so close to regaining my full health and yet still just out of reach. Her excitement at seeing the Lyme bacteria active and present reaffirms that I am closing in on destroying it. I laugh out loud at the inharmonious music my heavy bag of supplements makes as I walk through the parking lot to my truck. Devil's claw bangs noisily against the wormwood and horsetail leaf bottles, cat's claw and stinging nettle clang together like cymbals, and slippery elm, white willow, and other bottles with names I cannot pronounce tap each other softly like tambourines.

Nicole was not kidding when she said I would feel worse before I feel better. The Lyme bacteria puts up a good fight and makes me terribly uncomfortable while it tries to stop me from killing it. It does everything it can to maintain residence in my body and prevent eviction. It causes my limbs to twitch and flail, floods my mind with disturbing thoughts about death, and sends my blood pressure and heart rate sky high. I increase my dosage each day, pushing my body and mind to the limit, because I know this extreme discomfort is only temporary. I feel noticeably better two weeks later when the worst is over and the fog clears.

Dr. Nick and I have our last coaching call in February 2020. It is bittersweet saying goodbye to him, but we both know our time together has run its course. I tear up during our last hour together as I reflect on the progress I have made while knowing there is still more to do. He has been my Yoda, and I the diligent student thirsty for his wisdom. He educated me on the world of holistic healing, encouraged and challenged me, helped me become my own health advocate, and provided me with the confidence to heal all aspects of myself. He made himself available at a moment's notice and has been there for me in ways that no traditional Western medicine doctor has ever been. Now he reassures me that his door is always open and that I can reach out to him any time with questions.

Dan and I travel to Nashville for a joint bachelor-bachelorette party for one of his good friends from high school. I am tired, jumpy, and fatigued from this last round of supplements, but I participate in the festivities as much as I can while ordering salads and napping when necessary. I karaoke on stage and watch my friends ride a mechanical bull. We ride scooters from one destination to the next. We sample each other's drinks and jokingly laugh about Covid and germs as we catch glimpses of stern news anchors discussing potential shutdowns, travel restrictions, and masks. Everyone on Broadway in downtown Nashville is happy, living in the moment and enjoying the sunshine, and I feel blessed that I can do the same. Viruses, pandemics, and the upcoming election are worlds away.

CHAPTER 24

It's the End of the World As We Know It

MARCH 2020 – OCTOBER 2020

Schools are closed for the next two weeks. I have been nonchalant about the pandemic rumblings up until now, but I think it prudent to stock up on food at the grocery store in case things take a turn for the worse. I am shocked to find the shelves barren—bruised bananas, overripe cantaloupes, and sorry heads of wilted lettuce are some of the only produce remaining. Lone cans of dented nonperishables hide in the hard-to-reach places of dusty shelves, cowering there like lost children. The stores have been looted overnight, pillaged and plundered by desperate villagers during the zombie apocalypse. Two women argue loudly over the last package of toilet paper, and I am confused why paper goods are suddenly a hot commodity, as valuable as gold. We are only going to be housebound for two weeks, after all.

I am excited at the prospect of our family being home together for the next fourteen days. I envision mornings with no alarm clocks, savoring cups of coffee with Dan after a lazy breakfast, movie nights on the couch with cozy blankets and overflowing bowls of popcorn, and taking care of house projects that have been on our to-do list for months. This is going to be a mini staycation, a joyous time to reconnect with one another and stay up late playing Scrabble and Yahtzee.

Daily updates from the school district extend the closure time, first by days and then by weeks, until I reluctantly accept that schools will not be reopening at all for the foreseeable future. I turn into a teacher overnight and gain a newfound appreciation and respect for all the educators out there, for their tireless dedication and patience in molding the minds of our future generations. Remote learning for three children is challenging for everyone involved, and my patience wanes as quickly as a crescent moon.

Our house seems to shrink in between virtual classroom meetings while the pile of dishes in the sink and clutter of toys expand. I feel like the giant Alice in Wonderland stuck in the White Rabbit's house after consuming the "Eat Me" cake. We trip over each other and invade each other's private space. Our once idyllic staycation is now fraught with tension and annoyance at the tiniest thing—how we chew our food or brush our teeth, the sound of blowing noses like nails on a chalkboard.

To combat the monotony, we cut out shiny pictures from magazines and make colorful vision boards, spend hours placing tiny plastic gems onto sticky diamond art canvases, sprinkle the dining room table with 1,000 dusty puzzle pieces, and decorate the driveway in chalk rainbows all before noon. I am ready for the world to reopen. I long to stroll down the aisles of Target looking for nothing in particular and yearn for a few hours of uninterrupted silence to myself. Zoom and FaceTime keep us connected to friends and family but have lost their initial appeal of those first few weeks of quarantine when we were blissfully ignorant of what lay ahead.

Common Core elementary school math is much different from the math principles I grew up learning; the answer is still the same, but the deductive reasoning has changed. I try my best to help Everly understand simple addition and subtraction, the basics of multiplication, but rage slowly builds within me when the concepts don't click for her. Each time I repeat myself and start again from the beginning. I scribble in her notebook with such force that the pencil tip breaks and I give up on my subpar teaching skills.

Everly is in tears, and I hate myself for losing my temper and being the cause of her distress. We take a much-needed break from learning so we can both regroup. I lie in bed and sob as I mindlessly scroll through the sea of Facebook posts of creative parents who lovingly teach their kids with cute printouts and fun math tables, who come up with ways to make learning fun and a bonding experience. I furiously hurl my phone at the wall.

Out of control and scared, I notice symptom flare-ups that correlate precisely with the timing of my mental health going off the rails—joint pain, brain fog, anxiety, sleep disruption. Overcoming depression and chronic illness is like diving to the bottom of the ocean and then slowly making my way back up, being forced to stop at certain points to acclimate to the pressure change and perhaps having to go back down deeper before swimming up higher. This is one of those times when I must go down deeper and address the unresolved cause of my distress until the pressure dissipates, until I can safely swim back up to the surface.

I have learned so much about natural healing these past two years and how we are responsible for and in charge of our own health. I have choices. I have been making decisions for my health and I haven't been scared of getting sick and getting derailed. Covid is a positive year for me in terms of physical health. It certainly takes an emotional toll, but my mental state is stronger now, better equipping me to handle this in a constructive manner rather than in a self-destructive way.

Our society has become dystopian overnight. We are under strict government orders to stay home at all costs. Going out in public is frowned upon, but if you must, then a mask must be worn to protect our citizens from a virus that cannot possibly be contained, that moves unseen and undetectable like a silent assassin. Conspiracy theories are rampant, and I fall prey to this, getting sucked into the swirling whirlpool of the heightened political landscape, social media wars, bats from Wuhan, government control, and election fraud. People fight over toilet paper and gallons of milk through muffled words behind face shields and double masks, and I am appalled at how quickly we go from civilized to downright savages.

I'm angry that I spent these past few years healing myself and now the watchful eye of Big Brother is telling me that they know best, that my body is theirs for experimentation, that the only way to stay safe and do my part is to let them inject me with a vaccine. I am recalcitrant and disobedient, and I refuse to fall in line with the rest of the masked sheep. I defiantly show my full face during the height of the mask mandates. I get yelled at by some people as though I am a walking ball of Covid, while others pull their masks down, expose their mouth and nose as they walk by me, and give me a silent wink as though we are both in on a juicy secret. I attend church with a roomful of the unmasked as we smile largely at one another and sing loudly during worship, our germs commingling and fortifying our immune systems.

Although I am aware of and now understand the impact that thoughts can have on physical health, I am still in the infancy stages of taking action to reframe my perspective. The paralyzing effect of my mind chains me to my inner demons, and it takes every ounce of willpower to drown out the loud external noise. Making my mental health a priority right now is difficult when I am tethered so close to Dan and the kids, but it is imperative that I focus on this. I have not come this far just to come this far.

The gift of time has been handed to me on a silver platter; what I do with it matters more than ever. I am leading the way and setting an example for our children, and I want to create stability and normalcy in a world that is spiraling out of control. I know that these are crucial formative times for them, that their experience of this pandemic will largely mimic mine.

I control the controllable: the space between my ears. I rebelliously delete my Facebook account as the escalating political posts and online wars create further division among friends and our country. I refuse to compare my darkest moments to someone else's staged snapshot showcasing just how great their life is or how their family is embracing the pandemic in matching jammies and vats of hot cocoa. Tuning out the peripheral rumors and focusing on what works for our family, I slowly move from anger to acceptance. I adapt and embrace each day, taking satisfaction in knowing that if the only productive thing I accomplish in a day is making my kids smile by painting with them, then I have won the day.

Encouraging podcasts by Ed Mylett, Brendan Burchard, and Erwin McManus soothe my ears and my soul. Their passion is so strong it flows through my phone directly into me. I stop living in fear that my health will decline again and that our world will self-implode. I wake up every morning with faith foremost on my mind. I know that God has a plan, that everything will work out in due time. Daily affirmations à la Stuart Smalley seem silly but put me in a better frame of mind and force me to smile as I repeat, "I'm good enough, I'm smart enough, and doggone it, people like me!"

I reach for Islena like a lifeline, and her voice grounds me, reminds me of how far I have come, reassures me that I am more capable of reparenting myself than ever before. Our calls dwindle as my healing becomes a matter of being, rather than doing. It has happened so slowly that I didn't even notice it occurring, each incremental step building upon the next until the point where I started is barely recognizable. Just like Dr. Nick, she has taught me how to rely on myself, decrease my dependence on her, and stare at my shadow until I embrace her with love instead of run from her in fear.

CHAPTER 25

Bittersweet Symphony

NOVEMBER 2020 – FEBRUARY 2021

My return to physical health is almost complete, so much so that Dan and I commit to doing 75 Hard, a physical and mental toughness challenge. The rules are simple, but the execution is anything but. The 75 Hard program consists of two 45-minute workouts per day, to be completed at least three hours apart, and one must be outside, regardless of the weather. Each day, for 75 days, we must read 10 pages of an educational book, drink a gallon of water, follow a diet of our choosing, abstain from alcohol, and take a progress picture in the mirror. If we miss or forget any one of these items, the challenge clock resets to day one.

In my typical "go big or go home" mentality, I decide that the perfect time to start this is the day after the highly contentious presidential election, which seems fitting. Hopefully it will provide a welcome distraction from the chaos and pandemonium that is inundating our country. The Thanksgiving feasts, holiday parties, and celebratory toasts will test our resolve and strength, but doing this together is another testament of our commitment to bettering ourselves and our marriage.

My alarm clock buzzes at an ungodly hour each morning long before the winter sun rises low in the eastern sky and paints the horizon purple. I sleepily layer two pairs of pants and three sweatshirts under my long down parka to brave the subzero temperatures and glacial wind chills of the Midwest. A warm air front blows through Wisconsin for 18 hours, and I endure the torrential downpour it brings with it as water squelches between my toes. I slip and slide on the streets when they turn to ice the next morning. I slog through icy-cold slush in a raging blizzard until my feet are numb and step into a ditch as plow trucks thunder past. A car slowly creeps by, and the driver stops and cracks his window to ask if I am lost or need help. I laugh and tell him I am just out for my daily walk. I see the confusion on his face and know how ridiculous I must look to him—resembling the lumbering Stay Puft Marshmallow Man.

After a month, I arise before my alarm even goes off, and I look forward to the icy blast of chill air that greets me. These morning walks remind me of how far I have come, that with determination and grit I can overcome anything and that I am stronger than most. I am willing to do what others are not.

I do bicep curls with my gallon jug of water and jokingly discuss this with strangers when they undoubtedly comment, asking me if I seriously consume this in one day. Eggnog, holiday-themed cosmopolitans, and spiked cider are plentiful, and friends offer me large goblets of wine as they say, "It's the holidays! One drink won't hurt." I politely decline and say "cheers" with my club soda and lime. I realize that abstaining from alcohol is easier than I expect. My body thanks me each morning as I wake up clearheaded and refreshed. My diet does not require a great deal of modification, but instead of a gluten-free cookie for dessert, I opt for some fresh organic fruit. Reading before bed puts me in a sound mental state, and the progress picture of myself every morning when I feel the lightest is all the encouragement I need to keep going.

There is no built-in rest period and zero margin for error. Two workouts a day is certainly tiring, and the internal dialogue about whether to rest or complete my second workout gets louder the last three weeks of the program. I dig deep, remind myself once again of the connection between body and mind, that this is easy compared to what I have been through. Checking off each task at the end of the day provides a welcome sense of accomplishment and satisfaction. Our kids cheer us on, ensuring that we successfully complete the challenge. I am becoming a mother my children can be proud of.

My follow-up appointment with Nicole for biomeridian testing has been pushed back several months due to the pandemic, so I order more supplements and continue with the protocol she recommended for eight additional weeks. When I finally see her again, we embrace warmly, neither of us concerned with masks or distancing, and catch up on each other's lives as I get settled into the weathered armchair while Nicole taps away at her computer.

This round of biomeridian testing is shorter than my other appointments. When Nicole removes the electrode from my thumb for the final time and finishes typing up her notes, she turns to me with a big smile. "Sarah, this is incredible. Lyme bacteria are nowhere to be found, and I don't think it is because it's hiding beneath biofilm. Your body is truly healing!"

I jump out of the chair, grab her in a large bear hug, and shriek with joy. This is a triumphant win for both of us, reaffirming her knowledge of natural healing and my determination to overcome the beast of chronic Lyme. Although this is a relief, I know how thin the line is between the kingdom of the sick and the kingdom of the well and that I must stay alert and attentive to any future signs my body gives me, that remission is not promised forever and is a gift to be handled with extreme care.

I now sip San Pellegrino with two limes instead of champagne during our weekly baths as Dan and I reflect on and catch up on the chaos of each week. The brokenness inside has slowly been escaping, creating a lightness and levity that buoys me when dark thoughts and difficult moments arise.

My monthly cycle returns, intermittent and light at first then becoming as regular as clockwork. I am ecstatic at the cramping and bloating and welcome the sight of blood each month.

Dan and I celebrate my improving health with a trip to Punta Cana with six of our close friends. Our group floats in inner tubes around the lazy river as bartenders walk alongside and hand us glasses of water and piña coladas. We order plates of nachos from room service, eat soggy corn chips dripping in gooey processed cheese from the comfort of our patio lounge chairs, and throw olives at each other and try to catch them in our mouths. We play beach volleyball in the white sand, sarcastically ridicule each other's lack of skills, and laugh as the warm wind carries the ball in the wrong direction and into the frothy water. The live shows at night are better than I expect, and I scream for my brave (somewhat tipsy) friend who wanders up on stage to dance with the entertainers.

Late at night, we sit in a hot tub that feels like bubbling lava, the chlorine stinging the tiny cuts on our feet from seashells. We pass around a bottle of sickly sweet champagne, take a swig, and pass it to our left. Someone throws out the brilliant idea that we should strip down and run naked on the beach, and in a champagne-induced haze, we all agree. We splash in the waves and cackle at the absurdity of what we are doing. We feel completely uninhibited, wild, and free. The moon shines down upon us, illuminating both the calm water and our childlike giddiness.

I am alive and whole, my once-fragile body now strong, buoyed by the commingled salt water from the Atlantic Ocean and Caribbean Sea. I was running for so long from my life and now I am running for it, getting comfortable in my skin, in my own presence, in who I am. I am finally living again.

CHAPTER 26

Broken Halos

MARCH 2021 – JUNE 2021

    I attend church with Dan more frequently, and after trying out several different houses of worship, we eventually find our spiritual home in a nondenominational church that welcomes me as a Jew. While I do not consider myself religious, I have come back to faith and believe in God once again, my spiritual connection with a higher power restored. Before we got married, Dan was clear that he wanted to raise our children with a Christian upbringing, which I wholeheartedly agreed to. These roles are reversed from my childhood, as Mom took the reins and insisted on a strong religious foundation rooted in Judaism, which Dad agreed to with the caveat that we would also celebrate and be knowledgeable about his Catholic faith.

    My dear friend and neighbor Carol leads the women's Bible study and encourages me to join. As we read the book of Esther, I feel out of place as women confidently flip through the highlighted pages of their well-worn Bibles, yet also at home as the story of Purim is celebrated throughout the passages. Since I have no Bible of my own to follow along with, my thoughts wander back to the many hours of my youth spent in temple and Hebrew school discussing the same story of Esther. Warm memories rush in of making traditional Jewish pastries, rugelach and hamantaschen, with Grammy, and they comfort me. I say the Shema, the most essential prayer in all of Judaism, silently in my head, and jokingly wonder if I will be struck down by lightning for reciting Jewish prayers in church.

As women quote scripture, I sit in quiet reflection and talk to God. I forgive him for taking Mom and Mike too early and acknowledge that I would not be who I am today if they were still here. The theme of Esther is how to discover the presence of God when God appears to be absent, something I find extremely relevant to my current situation. I thank God for guiding me through illness, for loving me when I hated Him, for placing people like Carol and MK in my life when I needed them most, angels in plain sight. The inescapable longing that has tortured my soul for years dissipates as my renewed sense of faith grows.

I will never fit into anyone else's ideal spiritual box, and I am comfortable with this, unconcerned with the judgment of others. I am the only one to stay seated while the rest of the congregation takes communion, understanding full well that I know God just as much as they do. I teach my children how to light the Menorah and recite Jewish prayers with our Christmas tree as a backdrop. I stand firm in my own belief, knowing that it's OK to be different, that I have spent my entire life being different and hating it, and now I embrace it.

The shift in political power and uncertainty in our government causes intense chaotic upheaval as riots and protests break out daily amid voter and election fraud, accusations and acts of racism and hate, new variants of virus strains and vaccination requirements. Mask mandates lift overnight, as if the virus suddenly disappeared after the election. The girls and I skip to school with our faces fully exposed and smiling; I am filled with joy that they can breathe freely again and we are back in charge of our own health. The tissue-paper masks I bought for them were nothing more than defiant compliance that allowed them to attend school with the rest of their grade.

My father and brother, Matt, are convinced that our country is on the brink of civil war and encourage me to purchase firearms to protect my family. Dad would take me to the shooting range with him when I was only in middle school, wanting to ensure that I was comfortable with and knew how to shoot a gun should the need ever arise. My brothers and I would go to the outdoor skeet-shooting range in our later teenage years after Mom died. Their laughter and snickering at how my tiny frame bucked from the recoil of the 12-gauge shotgun fueled my determination to hit every clay pigeon as I widened my stance and braced my core to steady myself.

I placate Dad and Matt now by going to the shooting range again. I feel the cool weight of Sig Sauers and Glocks in my petite hand and marvel at the pinks and purples they come in now, looking more like toy guns than actual weapons. Dad and I put our protective headphones on, and I flinch at how loud the noise is inside the range, louder than I remember from years ago.

I close one eye as I pull the trigger with steady hands and completely miss the target, stumbling backward an inch as adrenaline courses through my veins. Dad laughs and yells muffled instructions at me as I square up again. The next shot hits the paper but just barely.

I remember my sixth-grade dream of being a police officer and Dad talking me out of it, scared of my small stature and the idea of his daughter fighting crime and redirecting my career choice to something safer. As I hit a bullseye, I try not to think about how Mike once pointed a similar-caliber gun at his own head.

As turbulent as the world is, I feel safe and protected amid the chaos. I trust that society will right itself in due time. I am not naïve about there being true evil in our world, however, I refuse to focus on this and let it consume me. The daily news would have enveloped me in grief and despair not long ago, but I now make the conscious decision to tune it out. I want to stay informed but not overly involved to preserve my sanity and health.

My goal is to provide a stable environment for my family, and our children flourish as Dan and I continue to put the time and effort into strengthening our marriage. We have the difficult conversations, and we are transparent with our kids about what is happening in the world as we reassure them that things will work out exactly the way they are supposed to.

I buckle my seatbelt tightly in the passenger seat of my truck as I teach Nolan how to drive, amazed that I already have a 16-year-old. I think about how young he still is, how there is so much for him to learn and experience. I know that I cannot possibly protect him forever and that our time together is limited. A twinge of jealousy coupled with anger hits me as 16-year-old Sarah shows up and whines about how unfair it is that Nolan has not had to deal with the enormity of pain and loss yet. I reflect upon the times when I have gotten frustrated with Nolan, and now I realize that it was rarely about him, that my reactions had more to do with my younger self still processing grief and loss. Parked in the garage after I bark orders at Nolan on how to turn the wheel, I apologize to him and explain that sometimes I get jealous that he has it so good and how I had to grow up faster than most teenagers did.

He drives us to the Department of Motor Vehicles the day of his road test for that glorious rite of passage that opens the door to an entirely new level of freedom. We check in with the surly worker who hands us a number and wait patiently in the cracked plastic chairs. Nolan points out a man doing pushups on the sidewalk, and I laugh it off and tell him that the DMV is always a great place to people watch, providing entertainment that rivals the Wisconsin State Fair.

A retired ex-Marine road examiner lumbers out from deep within the bowels of the government building, his biceps bulging and accentuating the tattoos that cover his arms. He calls Nolan's name, and Nolan turns to me in fear and eyes wide with terror. I chuckle, give his arm a squeeze, and tell him not to worry. Nolan trembles as they walk in formation to his pickup truck, and I pray that the steel-faced military man does not go too hard on him.

His road test allows me ample time to sit in silence with Young Sarah. I allow the memories to flood back, and I think about the day of my road test, how Grammy went with me because Mom was in the hospital dying. I drove to the hospital afterward and proudly showed Mom my new license, then counted down the minutes until I could leave the depressing room with its antiseptic scent that never could quite cover up the stench of death. I give Young Sarah a hug and let her know her pain is valid, but it is time to let it go. I remind her that life is not a competition, that Nolan will have different wounds to deal with and that she should be thankful he has not had to experience what she did. Nolan returns, and I embrace him with a bear hug before he smiles awkwardly for his license photo.

Many of the things I am doing today were completely unimaginable three years ago: working out twice a day, attending church, reparenting my inner child, standing firm in my beliefs and values. My walks at 5:00 a.m. in the cold darkness with nothing but my thoughts allow plenty of time for reflection and introspection and allow me to strengthen the laziest and most complacent muscle in my body—my mind. I speak to myself with kindness, understanding, and positivity, acknowledging the messy progress I've made and staying radically focused on the present moment. I can see clearer than I have in years. Examining my pain under a microscope and dissecting it bit by bit has unraveled the threads of mistruth that have kept me stuck and complacent.

The vast expanse of darkness in my heart is shrinking. The yearning for something unknown subsides, and as light pierces the horizon, it dawns on me that while I was busy searching for the missing puzzle piece, it was right in front of me all along. I am the missing piece.

CHAPTER 27

Mariposa

JULY 2021 – NOVEMBER 2021

I am drifting again, but this time back to myself. I am trusting my instincts more. The deep inner voice that had been silenced and shut down for years now speaks loudly, demands that I listen. More in tune with my body and mind than ever before, I succumb to what they tell me in any given moment. Lightness and ease encompass most of my days, and I enjoy a sense of belonging. I take up the space I deserve, owning my place in our chaotic world, and become firmly rooted in who I am. I lovingly embrace all the separate and distinct parts of me—the beautiful and the broken, the light and the shadow, the little girl, the lost teenager, and the 40-something-year-old mother and wife.

A routine MRI reveals that a small prolactinoma (a type of tumor that develops in the pituitary gland) has doubled in size over the past five years. While not pushing on my optic nerve yet, it may account for the constant headaches that still afflict me. Even though I share no genetic DNA with Mom, I panic. She died from a tumor on her pituitary gland.

Talking this over with Islena, she points out that because patterns are subconsciously passed down from parental figures, children learn and imprint by watching their parents, implying that illness is not always genetic or hereditary. I mull this over, angry that I may have manifested this by watching Mom's descent into fatal illness. Islena senses my thinking and helps me out of the trap of culpability and self-blame. No longer a victim of my past subconscious programming, I now have a choice over my reactions and thoughts. I choose positivity and grasp tightly to my newfound faith, knowing that everything will be OK. I seek out an endocrinologist who specializes in dealing with prolactinomas, and we devise a plan of action to shrink the tumor.

Dad falls ill with severe cardiac issues, and just like with Mom, my siblings and I take turns standing vigil over him at the hospital. I watch him dry heave into the garbage can. Wires stretch taut and IVs tug at his ashen skin as he bends over in the chair to retch out a few drops of saliva. Sixteen-year-old Sarah is immediately triggered, back in the ambulance with Mom, ready to detach and protect herself.

Islena's voice echoes in my mind and urges me to stay present and fully experience the deep well of raw emotion that crashes into me, and I come back to myself. I help Dad from the chair and into his hospital bed when the nausea subsides. He can barely maintain a conversation because he is so short of breath, but he talks about leaving the hospital and going home in between abnormal gasps for air. I hug him tightly and prop a pillow behind his head. His eyelids droop with exhaustion as I say goodbye, and the beeping monitors soothe him to sleep. He is a much better doctor than patient.

I think about the fragility of life as I get lost in the maze of hospital corridors. I pass a priest on his way to give last rites, and I am grateful that I am still on this side of the tenuous line between life and death. I allow the tears to fall, embrace the pain that slices through me, and ponder what life will look like without Dad.

We go to lunch a few months later when he recovers, and I hesitantly bring up a difficult yet necessary topic.

"Dad, we need to discuss what happens if you don't make it out of the hospital next time. I know you have a will and health-care directive, but I'd like to hear directly from you what your wishes are."

"If I ever get to the point where I can't wipe my own ass and you have to change my diapers, just leave me outside in the woods with a gun and walk the other way."

"Come on, Dad. I'm being serious."

"OK, OK. Your sister is my durable power of attorney for health care, so she knows what my wishes are regarding that. When I'm gone, I want you to take care of Candy, make sure she always feels welcome in our family."

"That's a given. Candy is as much a part of this family as anyone else. She's been a mother figure to me since I was sixteen."

Our dialogue is straightforward as though we are chatting about the weather, not tiptoeing around this somber subject with jokes or niceties.

"I want my funeral to be a celebration, for you to drink Bailey's and keep my memory alive with laughter at all the good times. I know most of your memories of Mom are of her being sick, but I hope you remember the good times with her as well, how she would do anything for you and your siblings."

Dad opens up and tearfully recalls the crushing devastation he felt when she didn't recognize him at the end, how he would pump her full of ever-increasing doses of Ativan to combat the night terrors and delusions. I always thought it was just me that she didn't recognize.

"Sarah, I'm so proud of your determination to find answers and get better. I know you had some dark days, probably darker than I imagined, and I'm just glad you're in a better place now. I wish you would have shared more with me so I could have supported you better."

"We both know that's not how our family operates. We have a history of remaining stoic in the face of adversity, maintaining that impression of strength even in the darkest of times. I know that this was necessary for us to move forward, but I think this is also one of our biggest downfalls."

"You're probably right. I didn't know how to talk to you kids about grief after Mom died, and none of you approached me to talk either. I'm sorry for that."

"There's nothing to apologize for. We did the best we could at that time. Now that we are all adults, I hope that we can have more authentic conversations, be vulnerable and honest with each other. It won't be easy, but I think that's the key to repairing the fractures in our family dynamic."

We stare into each other's tear-filled eyes and Dad nods, both of us knowing this conversation is a step in the right direction. I feel better equipped to handle grief than ever before.

Life is all about listening to the inner knowing that has always been with me but has been silenced for so long. I pay close attention to what my body and mind tell me. One day I eat gluten-free cookies and drift melodically into a sugar-coated ether and then the next I drink celery juice and hop on the Peloton for a ride with Cody or Alex. I lace up my dusty running shoes and hit the pavement, delight in the bliss of endorphins when my runner's high kicks in. A painful hip injury requiring surgery derails my half-marathon training, and I gracefully (begrudgingly) accept that long-distance running is no longer in my future. I refuse to push through the pain like I would have in the past.

I rest when necessary and continue to practice saying no to focus on my continued recovery. My healing is nonlinear, an everchanging process, enmeshing progression and regression, and it looks much different now than it did four years ago. The mental recovery has proven, by far, to be a more formidable obstacle than the physical recovery of chronic Lyme disease. I have taken control over what happens between my two ears. I accept my wins, and I forgive myself when I stumble upon old patterns that no longer serve me. A butterfly can never go back to being a caterpillar, and I am emerging from my cocoon.

CHAPTER 28

Fix You

SEPTEMBER 2021 – DECEMBER 2021

Word gets out around the gym that I am feeling better, and people I have not heard from in years as well as friends of friends reach out to tell me about their own mysterious symptoms: "I haven't been feeling like myself lately, but my bloodwork is all normal." "I've seen so many doctors and I'm starting to think that everything is all in my head." "My brain doesn't work like it used to." "I don't remember having a bullseye rash or being bit by a tick, but I spend a lot of time hiking in state parks."

We meet for coffee with collagen peptides in the tiny café of the gym lobby or for smoothies and protein powder at the organic grocery store or over the phone for those who are housebound. I listen to their all-too-familiar stories and sympathize with the physical symptoms that afflict them. I note the deep undertones of emotional wounding they gloss over and hold space when they tell me about the horrific abuse they encountered during their youth. I sit there and lighten the burden by sharing and holding their pain with them. I let them know they are seen and heard, that they are not crazy and can get better. But I'm also careful to set clear boundaries for myself to ensure my continued healing.

I relate to every word and feel relieved that I am at the tail end of my journey instead of at the beginning like they are, knowing they are going to go through arduous months of healing and dark nights of the soul before they get better. Most of them scoff when I mention the mental component, certain that no emotional baggage could possibly be contributing to their ailments. They are desperate to know what my secret is, what supplements I took and what protocol I followed, what magic recipe I concocted to reclaim my health.

Finding a way back to health is personal and intimate, and their path is not mine to walk. I leave them with a copy of Kelly Noonan Gores' book, *HEAL*, handwriting words of encouragement in the front cover and letting them know they can reach out to me for support.

An unintended consequence of getting sick is that my illness is helping others. Reading and hearing stories of others who have overcome insurmountable trials has provided me with a sense of connection and community throughout my recovery. Knowing that someone else has gone through a similar ordeal, felt the same emotions and symptoms, made me not feel so alone during those dark moments. Their stories of redemption inspired me to keep going, and now, in my final stage of healing, it is time to use what happened to me to help someone else.

Our conversations reinforce my reason and validation for sharing my story, for turning my pain into purpose, for helping the person I used to be. Illness made me bitter, resentful, and unrecognizable, however it was also the inciting change for who I was meant to become. My weakness was the channel through which God showed me my strength, where my best self grew out of my darkest place.

There are moments when I still doubt myself and question my wealth of knowledge on chronic Lyme disease. I tell myself that just because something worked for me does not mean it will work for someone else, that I must wait until my story is complete, for the last chapter when I will be completely mended and whole, before I can help others. And then I realize that I do not know what my last chapter will be until it is too late. The slow dawning of revelation seeps in as I think about the fact that if MK had not shared her story with me, I may not even be here today. This fuels me to keep going, extinguishes the lingering uncertainty, and propels me forward.

I am grateful for the gentle movement of my body in the crisp air before the rest of the world awakens. I watch the beauty of a pink and orange sunrise, see the way the light filters through the trees highlighting the floating particles suspended in air. The energy is palpable and charged with hope, and peace washes over me. I accept that my story will continue to change and evolve and that it's time to take advantage of today and seize the opportunity to fulfill my purpose now.

I celebrate my 42nd birthday in a rinky-dink town in Ohio with Dan and two of our friends. I enjoy every minute and laugh the entire time as our comfortable back-and-forth joking banter keeps us all in stitches. We have VIP passes to a concert and get to hang out with the band on their tour bus. Looking out at the crowd of concertgoers from backstage, Dan turns to me and says, "Who has it better than us?" Neither of us has truly been able to believe these words in years, but I am now beginning to wholeheartedly agree with him. We dance backstage under the full moon, drunk on life and a few shots of Fireball. Life is good.

Awakening from a deep sleep in the dead of night, I blink my eyes groggily as they adjust to the pitch black. I see the outline of a tall, shimmering, slender woman staring at me. I don't recognize her, but I feel no fear as she hovers there. I blink once, twice, three times, yet she remains steadfast, smiling, watching, protecting me. She slowly fades away as I move closer to Dan's warm body to ground me and then toss and turn until the first light of dawn. I feel more peaceful than I have in years. I know that this was a visit from the divine, and I feel secure knowing I am never alone.

The question I ask myself now is not whether I will survive; it is what do I want my life to look like after breaking and putting myself back together? Kintsugi is the Japanese art of repairing broken pottery by mending the areas of breakage with lacquer and powdered gold or silver, highlighting the imperfections instead of hiding them. It encourages fixing rather than discarding and represents the idea that we can heal and become stronger through our challenges and brokenness.

I focus on my beautiful children, my husband, my newly reclaimed health. I have learned that I can be two things at once: terrified and unafraid, unsure and certain, breaking apart and piecing myself back together. Getting sick saved me. It saved my marriage and my relationship with my children, but most important, my relationship with myself. Only when you are truly broken are you able to learn, grow, and gain perspective. I am better off broken than I ever was unbroken. I am covered in silver scars.

Epilogue

It has been almost four years since my recovery. Healing is not finite, and although there will always be setbacks, I am now equipped to tackle any physical or emotional difficulties that arise. I continue to learn and evolve. I talk myself through panic attacks and make myself feel hard feelings—I sit with them as they wash over me like an immense tidal wave of pain. Perhaps pain should be welcomed, not fought against, or ignored. It needs to be recognized just as joyful emotions are, for it has a purpose and is here for a reason.

I keep a strict gluten-free diet but no longer scrutinize ingredient labels or agonize over every bite of food—my juicer is pushed back and hiding in the dark corner of the cabinet. My supplements dwindle and then cease altogether, yet I know which ones to take if I feel rundown, which herbs will boost my immune system, and what the dosage should be based on the full moon and how long it has been since I last took them. The infrared sauna and coffee enema bucket sit unused, both such instrumental tools in my healing but now collecting dust like a first aid kit, used only in times of emergencies.

Most of the chapter titles of this book are songs that helped me through the darkest times in my life. There were times when music was my only friend, the pain in the melodic lyrics something I related to and the only thing that kept me going. It is difficult to remember what it was like to be so sick and in such a dark place, and I do not take this distance from it for granted. I know what a gift my health truly is, and I feel grateful each morning when I wake up.

Everly takes her first communion on the 26th anniversary of Mom's death, and I know my loved ones are there watching her, guiding all of us from another place yet still very much present. My rekindled relationship with God is personal and intimate, one that needs no clarification or explanation to others.

My past no longer defines me as I fully shed my victim mentality and walk in forgiveness instead of resentment. I take responsibility for who I am and for my missteps. I work together with Dan to create a marriage we enjoy being in and raise our children with faith and love. As Rumi says, "The wound is the place where the light enters you."

www.ingramcontent.com/pod-product-compliance
Lightning Source LLC
Chambersburg PA
CBHW020543030426
42337CB00013B/956